POSITIVE INITIATIVES FOR PEOPLE WITH LEARNING DIFFICULTIES

POSITIVE INITIATIVES FOR PEOPLE WITH LEARNING DIFFICULTIES

Promoting Healthy Lifestyles

Edited by
Roberta Astor and Karen Jeffereys

First published 2000 by
MACMILLAN PRESS LTD
Houndmills, Basingstoke, Hampshire RG21 6XS
and London
Companies and representatives throughout the world

ISBN 0–333–67208–9

A catalogue record for this book is available from the British Library.

This book is printed on paper suitable for recycling and made from
fully managed and sustained forest sources.

10 9   8   7   6 5   4   3   2   1
09 08 07 06 05 04 03 02 01 00

Editing and origination by
Aardvark Editorial, Mendham, Suffolk

Printed in Malaysia

Contents

CONTENTS

LIST OF TABLES AND FIGURES

Tables

Figure

NOTES ON CONTRIBUTORS

Roberta Astor MA, Cert in Further and Higher Education, RNT, RNLD, RGN, RMN
Staff Nurse, Portsmouth Healthcare NHS Trust.
Roberta has worked in Portsmouth since 1973, starting her career in learning disability nursing. She entered education as a clinical nurse teacher supporting students in learning disability practice. As nurse education moved to higher education, Roberta became a university lecturer. In this post, she was able to build on clinical expertise by developing a research interest in disabilities, with a particular focus on learning disabilities. Having been made redundant from her post as a university lecturer, Roberta has chosen to return to nursing practice. She now works for an NHS intensive care acute mental health unit, which serves the population of Portsmouth.

Sid Carter BA, RNLD, PGCEA, Adv Cert
Senior Lecturer, School of Health and Social Care, University of Portsmouth.
Sid is involved in an interprofessional course to prepare workers in the field of learning difficulties. His research interests are the neuropsychology of learning difficulties and primary care issues for people with learning difficulties.

Colin Goble RNLD/Dip MH, BA(Hons), MSc Applied Psychology (Learning Disabilities)
Lecturer in Learning Disabilities and Disability Studies, School of Management and Social Sciences, King Alfred's College, Winchester.
Colin formerly worked as a team leader in a residential service for people with challenging behaviour. His research interests include the links between health and challenging behaviours, the social model of disability and people with learning difficulties, and the history of services.

Karen Jeffereys State Registered Dietitian, MSc Applied Psychology (Learning Disabilities)
Chief Dietitian, Portsmouth Hospitals NHS Trust.
For 11 years Karen has managed a team of dietitians contracted to provide a specialist service to children and adults with learning difficulties in Portsmouth Healthcare NHS Trust. During this time, she has successfully initiated numerous service developments to improve the health of people with learning difficulties through diet and health promotion within the Trust.

Christine Jenkins MSc Applied Psychology (Learning Disabilities), PGDip, Dip RCSLT
Senior Lecturer, Department of Psychology, University of Portsmouth; Research Speech and Language Therapist, East Wiltshire Healthcare NHS Trust.
Christine divides her time between lecturing in the above MSc course, clinical practice and a 3-year investigation into the use of reading to develop the language skills of adults with Down's syndrome. Her interests lie in people with learning difficulties who also have hearing impairment, enabling choice and decision making for people with learning difficulties and the effectiveness of staff training in learning disability services.

Janet McCray RNLD, RNT, BSc (Hons), MSc
Principal Lecturer, Primary Care and Disability Studies, School of Health and Social Care, University of Portsmouth.
When working in practice, Janet has had a wide experience of working with people who have learning difficulties, largely in community settings. More recently, she has been involved in developing educational programmes in primary care and disability studies.

Richard Marler CQSW, BA (Hons), MSc Applied Psychology (Learning Disabilities)
Training and Development Officer, West Sussex Social Services.
In addition to researching the service needs of older people with Down's syndrome, Richard has a special interest in supporting local self-advocacy groups and involving service users with learning difficulties in training support staff.

Marilyn Nash RNLD, ITEC
Communication and Sensory Nurse, Portsmouth Healthcare NHS Trust.
Within various roles, Marilyn's practice has focused upon addressing the needs of people with learning difficulties who also have a visual impairment. Her innovative work has led to the specialist service taking a holistic view of the rehabilitation requirements of this group of people with complex needs.

Diana Sant Angelo BA (Hons), RNLD, Dip Couns
Community Nurse Team Leader, Portsmouth Heathcare NHS Trust.
Diana has 13 years' experience as a community nurse. Her interests include counselling the survivors of sexual violence, promoting sexual awareness and understanding, and working with men who have sexually offended.

Sue Shearman MSc Applied Psychology (Learning Disabilities), DipSw/DipHE, RSA Cert Hearing Therapy, RSA Cert Teacher of Lip Reading.
Care Manager and researcher in Oxfordshire.
Sue's main research areas and interest are in physical disability and dementia in young people. She has previously managed an audiology and hearing therapy service.

Professor Gregory Stores MA, MD, FRCP FRCPsych
Section of Child and Adolescent Psychiatry, University of Oxford Department of Psychiatry, Honorary Consultant in Neuropsychiatry, Oxfordshire Health Authority.
Gregory is head of a research programme into paediatric and psychiatric aspects of sleep and its disorders, and is the director of a sleep disorders clinic for adults and children. He has published over 100 articles on topics related to sleep disorders in children and childhood epilepsy.

Dr Rebecca Stores BSc (Hons), PhD, CPsychol
Research Psychologist, Section of Child and Adolescent Psychiatry, University of Oxford Department of Psychiatry.
Rebecca is currently conducting research into the prevention of and early intervention for sleep problems in young children with Down's syndrome. She previously worked at the Sarah Duffen Centre, a research establishment focusing on Down's syndrome, at

the University of Portsmouth. She has given numerous workshops and seminars to the parents of children with Down's syndrome and to professionals.

Dr Luci Wiggs BSc (Hons), Dphil
Research Psychologist, Section of Child and Adolescent Psychiatry, University of Oxford Department of Psychiatry.
Luci is involved in research into sleep, its disorders and treatments for these in children with developmental disabilities.

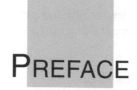

PREFACE

This book raises contemporary and controversial issues for care provision for people with learning difficulties. It aims to answer and challenge issues raised by policy and service provision, and should provide guidance to policy makers and service purchasers. Research-based chapters in this book break new frontiers and open interesting avenues for research reference. The book offers students, carers, researchers, service providers and purchasers stimulating material that has not been addressed in depth elsewhere.

The volume brings together a number of authors, with a direct service connection, who are innovative in their ideas and their approach to service delivery for people with learning difficulties. The authors come from a wide range of backgrounds, together providing a pool of information that should prove necessary and interesting for many practitioners or lay carers working with people with learning difficulties, as well as for researchers in the field. The changing market economy of care demands a broad knowledge and education base from all involved in care provision for people with learning difficulties. This volume provides information to direct both practice and service change.

The overall aim of the book is for each chapter to discuss an area relevant to achieving 'Health for All' for people with learning difficulties. It combines practice, research and an analysis of sociopolitical approaches to meeting health needs.

In Chapter 1, Astor and Jeffereys reflect upon the health services in historical terms and review the approach used to apply those contemporary policies and strategies aimed at improving the nation's health. They discuss possible strategic direction and argue the need for change in order to improve the health of people with learning difficulties.

The discussion of history and contemporary issues is continued in Chapter 2. Here, Carter provides an insight into processes of health care delivery, one which arises from examining the derivation of the philosophy and practice of primary health care. This is applied to the social context of people with learning difficulties receiving primary health care, in order to argue that many are systematically disenfranchised and disempowered. Evidence is presented that professionals can effect the progression to good-quality primary health care for people with learning difficulties.

Chapters 3–11 take a practice- and/or research-based look at specific health areas. Some describe actual practice, while others debate service delivery. Chapter 3 describes the experience of using the Look After Yourself (LAY) model, for enabling healthy lives, with people with learning difficulties. An account is given of the LAY programme, outlining seven programmes which were run in Portsmouth. This overview includes adaptations to the core model for the three components of exercise, relaxation and health topics. Although it has not been evaluated, the authors highly recommend this model.

Sant Angelo, in Chapter 4, focuses on nursing practice, addressing the emotional and sexual health needs of people with learning difficulties. These needs are linked to health issues that focus on human immunodeficiency syndrome, sexual health and mental illness. The role of the community learning disability nurse working in partnership with service users is described.

In Chapter 5, Goble uses a case study approach to demonstrate how a participatory dialogue between practitioners and service users can enable an escape from 'iatrogenic illness'. The work of a residential team using Shared Action Planning and Gentle Teaching Approaches exemplifies how entering into a natural dialogue with service users can empower them to achieve physiological and psychological health. This theme continues in many chapters, McCray (Chapter 6) advocating a partnership model for supporting women with learning difficulties during the antenatal period. She also makes suggestions that will help both potential mothers and midwifery staff in building relationships.

Sensory impairment is included in a list of health problems and disabilities more commonly experienced by people with learning difficulties. Nash's innovative work with people who have visual and learning difficulties proposes many ways forward for both residential and service development (Chapter 7).

Jenkins and Shearman's chapter on hearing impairment addresses service delivery needs to achieve health gain targets in this area.

Sleep problems are an often overlooked cause of considerable stress in families with a child with learning difficulties, and are therefore detrimental to health. In Chapter 9, Stores, Wiggs and Stores briefly introduce the topic of sleep problems and their effect on both the child and the family. Suggestions are made for improving currently available services that support children and families.

Marler (Chapter 10) proposes that service models are needed that respond appropriately to the needs of people with Down's syndrome who develop Alzheimer's disease. Recommendations for services are drawn from an examination of the Down's syndrome–Alzheimer's disease connection, with particular reference to diagnosis and care approaches. A small-scale study is described, which considers the service needs of this group as seen by families and care professionals.

In Chapter 11, Jeffereys examines quality issues related to one aspect of food service for people with learning difficulties living in residential care. The author reviews international and national practice, including two small-scale pieces of research and local developments. A spiral audit model describes how service users and providers can work together to produce comprehensive nutrition standards within local quality structures.

Finally Premise for Possibilities (Chapter 12) summarises the theme of the book in terms of inclusion in quality services. The learning disability nurse is focused on as the key person to coordinate health services. Three nurses give their own views and provide case studies on how they have improved health provision to their clients.

Specific mental health issues are addressed here by Marler, Sant Angelo and Yerbury, but the broad issue of mental health and challenging behaviour is not discussed. This book seeks to raise concerns not highlighted by *Our Healthier Nation* (DoH, 1998) and recognises that literature is rapidly emerging to address the areas of mental health and challenging behaviour needs for people with learning difficulties (Bigden and Todd, 1993).

An area that has been highlighted in some but not all chapters is that of enabling people with learning difficulties to access health information. There is, however, implicit within each chapter the opportunity not only to develop or improve services, but also to make information accessible. Further reference to Greenhalgh's (1994) report brings together the 'diverse aspects of health, information and learning difficulty' (p. 2). Like Greenhalgh, the authors continue to share knowledge and practice but emphasise that organisational change must occur in order to ensure that the correct services are commissioned in the future.

References

Bigden, P. and Todd, M. *Concepts in Community Care for People with a Learning Difficulty.* (Basingstoke: Macmillan, 1993).

Department of Health. *Our Healthier Nation: A Contract for Health.* A consultative paper. (London: Stationery Office, 1998).

Greenhalgh, L. *Well Aware, Improving Access to Health Information for People with Learning Difficulties.* (Anglia: NHS Executive, 1994).

ACKNOWLEDGEMENTS

The editors wish to acknowledge the time and commitment given by the contributors, staff and people with learning difficulties who have made this book possible. Special thanks also to Carol Holden RNLD, Team Leader; Amanda Yerbury RNLD/RMN, Community Nurse; and Kathryn Curtis RNLD, Team Leader, Learning Disability Division, Portsmouth Healthcare NHS Trust, for permission to use their case histories featured in Chapter 12.

1

INTRODUCTION

Roberta Astor and Karen Jeffereys

Health opportunities

There is a myth in the history of British service provision for people with learning difficulties that the model of services, particularly those services provided by the NHS has been a medical one. This myth arose from labels attached to parts of the services. People lived in 'hospitals', staffed by 'nurses' and managed by medical superintendents – a socially devalued way of life that attached stigma to people with a learning difficulty. Despite the lack of many requisites for good-quality lifestyles, it could be assumed that the standard of care for maintaining physical health would be high. However, this was not so. Naming the large institutions 'hospitals' provided a socially acceptable means of segregation. Little medical care was provided to promote good health: the doctors were psychiatrists, not experts on the management of medical problems. Nurse training did not start to reflect changes from custodial care until the late 1950s. Registered nurses were thin on the ground for many years, the wastage rate from training was alarming, pay was low, and the hospitals were not attractive career bases (Bendal and Raybold, 1969).

Given this state of affairs, the physical health of people with learning difficulties was neglected. Indeed, when individuals were ill, they were unlikely to receive vital medical care as either the symptoms were attributed to their 'subnormality' or it was assumed that the hospital they lived in would provide the necessary care. It seems more appropriate to call the model 'death making' than medical. People with learning difficulties did not receive a high standard of medical care when they were physically ill, and this detoxified death making also excluded health promotion.

The advent of community care policies, which are actively closing hospitals for people with people with learning difficulties, is seen by the Royal College of General Practitioners (RCGP) as a possible source of problems for primary health care. Community care can be hailed as a new idea for service provision if it is forgotten that the majority of people with learning difficulties have always lived in the community. A substantial number of individuals have also escaped the medical model, and not because they have avoided institutionalisation.

Rodgers (1994, p. 11) cites evidence from studies undertaken in Britain, America and Australia to make the case that 'The health care needs of people with learning difficulties living in the community are in danger of being ignored.' Meehan and Moore (1995) found that most health promotion failed to meet the needs of people with a learning difficulty, and considered them liable to encounter problems in using mainstream health screening services. Meehan facilitated the development of a health screening service run by specialist community nurses. The screening revealed many previously undetected and treatable conditions, which could have been detected by general practitioners (GPs) and were likely to have been preventable given appropriate health education.

The Health of the Nation strategy document for people with learning difficulties claimed that this group of people:

> use health services less often than the general population. Too often, treatable illness is undetected until it has progressed to a stage where treatment is less effective. (DoH, 1995, p. 14)

Furthermore:

> Few primary care teams have the specialized skills to offer a complete service to people with learning disabilities. (DoH, 1995, p. 17)

According to Howells and Barker (1990), GPs lack training and experience in dealing with people with a learning difficulty. Stein (1996) has shown that GPs themselves have differed in their response to wanting more training. Possibly because of this lack of experience, some doctors appear to respond negatively to this client group and omit to offer them the same medical treatment as the rest of the general public. People with learning difficulties may not recognise or report the symptoms of ill health. In some cases, communication and cognitive difficulties cause problems with health screening. The RCGP considers that there is an enormous need for people with learning difficulties to have specialist help in overcoming communication problems.

2

Where people with learning difficulties can recognise symptoms of illness and are able to describe them, they may rely on their carers to support their use of doctors. Carers could, however, be elderly and unable to support their relative effectively, or may feel that the condition is not severe enough to merit consulting a doctor.

This disturbing evidence is compounded by the possibility that people with learning difficulties have a 'higher than average incidence of ill health and disability' (NHSME, 1993, p. 10). Similarities between people with learning difficulties and people in the lower social classes can be drawn with regard to social conditions such as income and diet: 'People may rely on pre-prepared food from canteens and fast-food outlets' (DoH, 1995, p. 20). Access to resources for making lifestyle changes are limited. It is hard for many reasons for people with learning difficulties to access the use of local leisure centres and family planning clinics, for example. The reasons can be economical, attitudinal (on the part of carers) or skills based.

The Department of Health (1991, p. 105) has reported 'a persistent gap between death rates among manual and non manual classes', said to be caused by a variety of influences. It has been argued that people in lower social classes choose to ignore healthy lifestyle opportunities. The counter-argument emphasises the need to alter social conditions and provide access to lifestyle changes via informed choice and appropriate services. Community care policies for people with learning difficulties that acknowledge principles of social role valorisation would agree with this counter-argument.

Health information

A 1995 survey by the Health Education Authority (HEA, 1995) found limited health promotion resources for people with learning difficulties, except in the area of sexuality, human immunodeficency virus (HIV) and acquired immune deficency syndrome (AIDS). Morton (1995) reports that it can be hard to provide education to promote the sexual health of people whose relationships go unrecognised. She also asks how people with communication difficulties can acquire condoms when they do not want their carers to know they are doing so.

People with learning difficulties may not be able to use health education to make informed decisions about their own health. In the words of the DoH, 'much of the age and sex-specific health care publicity material produced each year fails to reach its intended audience. It is not much help to those who cannot read and may not use language, and whose carers are in a different age group' (NHSME, 1993, p. 16).

Health politics

The RCGP states that the words 'learning difficulty' appear to diminish the seriousness of the issues in this area. The 1990 NHS and Community Care Act created an internal market of purchasers and providers of care, the funding structure of this market dividing health and social care. This was in conflict with World Health Organisation (WHO) principles, which do not define health solely within the health sector. 'Health promotion represents a mediating strategy between people and their environments', and 'the need for change in the ways and conditions of living in order to promote health' (Naidoo and Wills, 1994, p. 76) is recognised.

It could be argued that the move from institutions to community care promotes health for people with learning difficulties. There is well-documented evidence, however, to show that living in the community does not equal access to and participation in the community. The question 'Does the community care or even exist?' still needs to be asked.

Wide gaps occur in health status between different groups within as well as between countries. To address this, the WHO advocates the promotion of good health as part of the whole social and economic policy of a country, rather than changes being sought in health service delivery. The WHO notes the health service consumer as feeling 'that the health services and the personnel within them are progressing along an uncontrollable path of their own' (Rifkin and Walt, 1986, p. 561). Western capitalist society has never valued people who are not seen as enhancing the economic health of society; hence, circumstances for people with learning difficulties are unlikely to improve without a radical change in political will.

Unfortunately, despite WHO statements apparently supporting empowerment and advocacy, the underlying principles of Health For All by the Year 2000 are 'the attainment of all citizens of the world by the year 2000 of a level of health that will permit them to lead a socially and economically productive life' (Ewles and

Simnett, 1995, p. 13). While a reduction in the inequality of health is a key WHO criterion for assessing progress, the value base for the measurement of equality and inequality still militates against social role valorisation for people with learning difficulties. It is unlikely that social role valorisation can be attained by people with learning difficulties without major social transformation. The document *Our Healthier Nation* (DoH, 1998a) could have given impetus to achieving social role valorisation had the divide between health and social care been removed. The existence of this divide means that there is little chance of empowerment and participation for people with learning difficulties in achieving better health. Social role valorisation is not just about individual roles being valued. A valued social role can protect a person, and research shows that it certainly enhances the likelihood of attaining better health care; if that person is labelled as belonging to a devalued social group, however, he or she remains at risk. Social role valorisation is therefore about valuing the social role of people with learning difficulties as part of society as well as their individual roles.

Government policy and strategies

The New NHS (DoH, 1997a) and *Our Healthier Nation* (DoH, 1998a) aim to improve the health of the UK through 'modernisation' and forming a 'contract for health', by:

- improving the health of the population as a whole by increasing the length of people's lives and the number of years people spend free from illness
- improving the health of the worst-off in society, and narrowing the health gap (DoH, 1997, 3.10).

Together, these documents promise equity and quality services. For people with learning difficulties, this could improve access to, and treatment from, all health services.

Yet the criteria for developing these strategies take no specific account of people with learning disabilities. There is a need for government statements requiring Primary Care Groups (PCGs) and Health Action Zones (HAZs) to be sensitive to the needs of people with learning disabilities. (Mencap, 1998, p. viii)

5

The DoH are to pursue a new deal for people with learning difficulties (DoH, 1997). However, Gates (1998, p. 1) asks whether 'these new initiatives really contribute to, and promote the health and well being of, learning disabled people and their families' The government has acknowledged that they are a disadvantaged group of people who less frequently use services, also receiving poorer quality services. Accordingly, two publications and a cassette, *The Healthy Way* (DoH, 1998b) and *Signposts for Success* (Lindsey, 1998), have made recommendations for good practice. These documents set out expectations for service users, providers and purchasers in terms of what should be achieved in health care for people with learning difficulties.

Gates (1998, p. 2) warns against complacency posing the question:

Given that there already exists guidance for purchasers and commissioners of health and social care, why should citizens with learning disabilities believe that the new guidance outlined earlier will address the current inequity they experience regarding their health status, and the health service provided to them?

Certainly, there is little evidence of strategic planning in order to set goals inherent to statements such as 'there is also a need for well planned, comprehensive specialist services to be available to people with learning disabilities and their families (DoH, 1997b).

The New NHS (DoH, 1997a) aims for primary care Trusts to commission services for their local population. Does this include the specific needs of people with learning difficulties? Will the NHS executive prompt health authorities (HAs) to question this? It is interesting to note that although *Signposts for Success* (Lindsey, 1998) clearly has a primary care focus, there is a danger of commissioning details distancing learning disability services still further from primary care. Mencap (1998, p. 21) notes that:

The new process of primary care planning and commissioning through Primary Care Groups presents opportunities for people with learning disabilities, providing there is adequate representation of their interests, both through the Health Improvement Programmes (HImPs) and in the membership of PCGs.

Learning disabilities services certainly are expected to be commissioned not through primary care Trusts (Lindsey, 1998, 5.14) but through some other form of provision. It is suggested that specialist

Trusts might be formed, or alternatively specialist learning disability services could be provided by community health Trusts. Mencap (1998, p. 36) supports the notion of learning disability services being 'placed within primary and community care Trusts rather than mental health Trusts'.

Thus, the philosophy of *Our Healthier Nation* and *The New NHS* provides an opportunity to focus on the health of people with learning difficulties in order to create strong national strategies and networks alongside the appropriate local learning disability service structure. Discussions have inevitably taken place through multi-agency conferences to discuss policy issues (Community Care Development Centre, 1997). These provide a forum to hear from, and exchange views with, people who use and provide services. So far, however, forums have not been given the true weight necessary to see a positive change. A sceptic will wonder where the information from these conferences goes, and what systems exist to inform future policy and practice.

While considering this and the consultation questions asked in *Our Healthier Nation*, a number of potential weaknesses can be identified for people with learning difficulties. In order for these to be overcome, three issues need to be addressed. First, national organisational structures specific for people with learning difficulties must be established. Second, national communication networks accessible to all should be developed in order to disseminate good practice, research and audit. Third, systematic data collection on the morbidity and mortality of people with learning difficulties should be centrally collated in order to evaluate health outcomes.

Our Healthier Nation clearly aims to target the health of people marginalised by financial, social class, geographical and environmental factors. It gives clear direction on the four main health targets. However, it suggests that, in some areas, purchasers may choose to focus locally upon vulnerable groups of the population:

> In order to address the health needs of specific groups of people whose health is of particular concern, local strategies might address the needs of different minority ethnic groups, homeless people, single parents, socially isolated people, people with learning disabilities, people on low income or refugees. (DoH, 1998a, p. 81)

People with learning difficulties will, however, require more than just a mention if they are truly to be considered within local priority target setting frameworks. Vigorous positive discrimination is necessary if health changes are to occur nationally for people with learning difficulties. The Mental Health Foundation (1996, p. 8) has recommended that 'The Government should establish an independent Task Force for People with Learning Disabilities to investigate and report on key issues at ministerial level'. A national task force for people with learning difficulties could centrally coordinate and implement the strategy with special emphasis on meeting their needs. Such a task force could itself be charged with planning how these needs could be met within the overall strategic framework. The authors suggest potential roles and functions for the national task force (Table 1.1). It could form the natural, national organisational link between the DoH, service users, providers and purchasers.

Table 1.1   Potential roles/functions of a task force for people with learning difficulties

- Plan strategic direction specifically for the health needs of people with learning difficulties
- Develop tender specifications in order to establish a publicly accessible national communication network
- Coordinate a national directory of examples of good practice, such as projects that encourage and foster local community action
- Coordinate research/audit
- Develop specifications or checklists, for example a national contract for each of the four areas for people with learning difficulties – to be used by the Department of Health and purchasers (heatlh authorities) when considering all HImPs.
- Issue directives that all HImPs must formally report on whether and/or how they intend to meet the needs of people with learning difficulties
- Systematically identify those HImPs which neither address nor meet the needs of people with learning difficulties. Collate the unmet needs and use them for future planning/research/audit
- Respond to those HImPs which do not meet the needs of people with learning difficulties by informing the planners of other good practices and resources that could be implemented
- Provide information to HImPs on networking arrangements, for example local joint planning groups (LJPGs)
- Organise the collation of national morbidity and mortality data in the four target areas

HImPs = health improvement programmes.

Such a national task force would form the centre of national planning for people with learning difficulties, but it relies on a formally structured local focus: the local joint planning groups (LJPGs). *Signposts for Success* (Lindsey, 1998, pp. 7–8) clearly outlines the way in which LJPGs should work in partnership. However, national strategic planning should coordinate stages of working over a set number of years. Table 1.2 suggests such an approach.

The membership and roles of the LJPGs would need to be specified by the task force in order to ensure that key people from all agencies responded appropriately. LJPGs form the group that promotes local quality services for people with learning difficulties. Their role must include the dissemination and collation of information as directed by service users and the task force. They should be responsible for routinely accessing information from other districts and similarly sharing their own experiences through established national networks. Although *Signposts for Success* (Lindsey, 1998) has made a positive mark in setting out good practice guidelines, its principles now need to be supported by one lead body to communicate success. The emphasis must be on information flowing naturally through nationally established links in order to inform people up, down and across organisational structures.

Table 1.2   Strategic approach

First stage	Second stage
Support:	Help:
• the establishment of LJPGs	• LJPGs to determine local priorities using valid methodology
Setting up:	Ensure:
• systematic data collection	• all systems comprehensively communicate via national networks
• service user opinion	• the use of HImPs to identify areas of unmet need
• national channels of communication	

LJPG = local joint planning group; HImPs = health improvement programmes.

Prioritising key targets

The 1998 DoH strategy prioritises four key target areas – heart disease and stroke, cancer, mental illness, and accidents – these being identified as major causes of premature death or adverse effects.

Turner and Moss (1996) reviewed the issue of whether the key target areas of *The Health of the Nation* (DoH, 1992) were relevant to people with learning difficulties. They reviewed the evidence on mortality and risk factors, and concluded that the key areas were appropriate. However, the research reviewed does not reflect trends in mortality. The mortality trends of people living in a Bristol institution over a 50-year period (Carter and Jancar, 1983) show an increase in the number of carcinomas and sudden deaths, although respiratory disease continues to be the major cause of death. Turner and Moss suggest that other areas, for example sensory impairment and dental disease, also need to be prioritised for people with learning difficulties, concluding that *The Health of the Nation* only 'partially reflects the health priorities for this group' (Turner and Moss, 1996, p. 446). As this health policy addressed the same areas as *Our Healthier Nation*, Turner and Moss' conclusions would remain valid. However, respiratory disease as the major cause of death also needs to be prioritised.

Public health research provides the basis for health targets and priorities, yet local health targets may be set without taking the health needs of people with learning difficulties into account. It is clearly time to improve data collection on the health of people with learning difficulties. Trends in mortality and morbidity need to be more clearly defined in terms of age groups and actual disease. For example, the number of deaths from carcinoma was seen to have risen from one to 22 per year in a 50-year period (Carter and Jancar, 1983). Further statistical data, for example the types of cancer and age and sex trends, are now needed in order to plan effective action and services. If these were linked with the type of accommodation, it would form an excellent picture of the trend of a particular cancer and how moving from institutions to the community might have impacted upon mortality and/or morbidity. Such statistical review is beyond the scope of this publication because it requires national cooperation and a focus on gathering together unpublished data regarding the health trends in key target areas.

Such an analysis would underpin a true health strategy for people with learning difficulties. Thus, further statistical evidence is required in order to measure health gains for people with learning difficulties. There are concerns that, within the limited resources available, other areas of health promotion or health care may be marginalised or undervalued. Without data, it will be impossible to evaluate whether more or fewer health needs are being met.

Our Healthier Nation has chosen key targets that would seem to agree with some of the mortality and morbidity risks for people with learning difficulties, but are the routes for delivering health the best?

Routes to delivering health

Our Healthier Nation (DoH, 1998a) has chosen three key routes – healthy schools, healthy workplaces and healthy neighbourhoods – through which to channel change. This is a fine strategic approach except for those who are socially excluded by attending special schools or being unemployed, or who lack appropriate community presence, as is the situation for many people with learning difficulties.

Healthy schools

The emphasis on the national curriculum is currently a major barrier in special schools in terms of teaching healthy lifestyles.

Schools will require a range of evaluated, healthy lifestyle resources for children with learning difficulties with different abilities. Such an approach in school could then be followed by a lifelong learning approach, which should be provided by higher and further education establishments as well as traditional adult education services. It would be necessary to develop appropriate evaluated resources and course curricula for adults with learning difficulties. Pathways for educational attainment and development should be organised using the school curriculum as the building blocks.

Courses and lessons on healthy lifestyles do exist but most seem to be independent, repetitive and *ad hoc*, not always building on current skills. The National Vocational Qualification (NVQ) framework may have much to offer in this area. A healthy lifestyle curriculum should be planned so that people with learning difficulties could work systematically from childhood to adulthood at each individual's ability, age and pace. Personal competences portfolios could effectively link with the NVQ framework in order to enable lifelong learning. If such a curriculum were developed, teachers could easily share personalised resources, methods and outcomes. Easy access to such educational information should be made available via nationally and internationally linked channels of communication set up by the task force.

Healthy workplaces

Government policy acknowledges that a lack of employment and low income can adversely affect people's health. *Our Healthier Nation* (DoH, 1998, p. 17) states that 'being in work is good for your health. Joblessness has clearly been linked to poor physical and mental health.' The Welfare to Work programme aims to support people back to work. Most people with learning difficulties are unemployed, attending day services or in work that is devalued either by its social status or by unacceptably low pay. There is a need to examine the Welfare to Work programme, and any other government strategy aimed at promoting health by enabling better living standards through employment, to ask whether the needs of people with learning difficulties are being addressed. Any local initiatives, such as schemes aimed at people aged 25 and over who have been unemployed for more than a year should also include people with learning difficulties. These initiatives could link with lifelong learning educational approaches.

The Mental Health Foundation (1996, p. 82) recommends a government 'review of the overall effect of a range of social security benefits on housing, training and employment for people with learning disabilities'. It strongly endorses supported employment, in which work preparation is undertaken to help in finding a suitable job and gradually support is given to the individual to ease him or her into independent work performance. While supporting people into employment is a costly exercise, it can, when measured against longterm day centre provision, prove cost-effective.

The Disability Discrimination Act (1995) may aid employment opportunities for people with learning difficulties by putting the onus on employers (DfEE, 1996) to justify reasons for not offering employment and to make 'reasonable' adjustments to enable employment for disabled people. The Mental Health Foundation (1996, p. 38) calls for 'some of the benefits which people derive from a job, namely an income, social interaction and meaningful occupation during the day' to be available for people with learning diffi-culties whose multiple and complex disabilities are likely to exclude them from employment. This creates a need specifically to target day services, training centres and further education colleges in order to incorporate healthy lifestyle packages effectively, otherwise the message of healthy lifestyle choices via the workplace will not reach all adults with learning difficulties.

Healthy neighbourhoods

Approaches recommended by *Our Healthier Nation* for achieving healthy neighbourhoods embody familiar concepts for learning disability services. Community presence and social participation (O'Brien, 1987) form part of service ideology as targets to achieve for service receivers, yet social exclusion remains a major issue for people with learning difficulties. The Mental Health Foundation (1996, p. 70) wants a national public information exercise mounted to 'correct the false image of learning disability that exists widely in our society and causes public prejudice and rejection to occur'.

The *Signposts for Success* (Lindsey, 1998) document considers that all people with learning difficulties should live in their own homes and pursue ordinary lifestyles wherever possible. A high level of health needs, physical disability and infirmity caused by ageing are not reasons to exempt people if staff competence and skills are appropriate. The target of healthy neighbourhoods for people with learning difficulties should be addressed when placing people with learning difficulties in the community. *Signposts for Success* suggests avoiding placements which separate people from their friends and families. Placing too many people in one locality should also be avoided. The proximity of services for other groups of potentially socially devalued people can lead to 'ghettoisation' and make inte-gration into a neighbourhood more difficult.

Choice is a service accomplishment, which should be applied as part of achieving a healthy neighbourhood for people with learning difficulties. Every effort must be made to support participation by the person moving home in checking out potential future neigh-bourhoods and accommodation. It is sensible for everyone to check community facilities, crime rates, what the neighbours are like, health and education provision and any other pertinent factors before deciding to live in a particular place. It is also normal to consider whether the house you might move into suits your needs.

People with learning difficulties should be able to make decisions about where they want a home rather than have that choice made for them for economic reasons.

Tregelles (1998, p. 8) calls for 'a comprehensive housing strategy for people with special needs', asking the government to ensure that all agencies are talking to each other and that services are coordinated. She says that this is the only way to guarantee people the enjoyment of their own homes and to prevent the drive for the inclusion of disabled people into society grinding 'to a startling halt'.

Marketing

How can these key routes be achieved? Will good practice be disseminated nationally? Without exception, all agencies and service users will need to be involved through LJPGs working alongside initiatives in the HImPs.

Previous health strategies, for example *The Health of the Nation* (DoH, 1992), focused upon the needs of people by publishing a strategy for people with learning disabilities (DoH, 1995). This booklet was written primarily for purchasers of health and social care and was distributed by the DoH through regional health commissions and an out-of-date network list. However, the intent that it should be 'useful to GPs and other health service providers, to other providers, and to families' (Simpson, 1995, p. 19) seems to have fallen short as the booklet was extremely difficult to obtain. It lacked strategic distribution and was not nationally marketed through appropriate professional and carer channels, for example learning disability journals, *Target* (*The Health of the Nation* briefing sheet) and carers' forums.

The booklet stimulated three conferences in autumn 1995 (at the Hester Adrian Research Centre, East Berkshire NHS Trust and St George's Hospital Medical School). All informed participants about the health needs, but discussion led neither to a coordinated and shared approach nor to a strategic national approach. *Signposts for Success* (Lindsey, 1998) has taken the steps to provide information, but it will need vigorous marketing, along with published plans and national communication networks, to reach those who need it. Without these, the responsibility lies entirely with the individual service users, clinicians, small groups or localities to interpret and then demand or provide informed quality services.

The notion that commissioners 'may need to facilitate the development of information systems or of information gathering and analysis' (DoH, 1998a, p. 13, 2.31), as well as the checklist for Action (p. 15), will lead to introspective services unless it is linked with a strong national network. The document sets out the types of response (p. 12, 2.30) needed to meet the demands for good-quality information. It acknowledges the diverse, idiosyncratic and fragmented nature of some information, its incompleteness and inaccuracies, and the need to share current experiences.

Specific considerations

Without a doubt, we should ensure that people are able to choose, access and be supported to lead healthy lifestyles. However, health promotion needs to be targeted carefully. Consideration should be given to the individual's health status because what is one person's medicine may be another's poison.

Health strategies have traditionally focused upon the individual making informed choices and being able to act accordingly to change his or her lifestyle. However the issue for many people with learning difficulties is having the opportunity and skills to express their choice. People need information and skills to be able to make judgements about the choices available to them. Resources have to be available to support this work, and the HEA have produced a resource catalogue specifically aimed at the needs of people with learning difficulties (HEA, 1995). This needs to be regularly updated.

As in all health promotion, care must be taken when interpreting general health messages for the individual. Take diet as an example. National dietary targets should be interpreted with caution in order to avoid compromising people who are emaciated, have feeding difficulties or have high energy requirements because of constant activity. In contrast, obesity is often focused upon as an area of health need. It is, however, obvious that the type of treatment and nutrition education available to the public has had little impact, as the number of obese people continues to rise (DoH, 1995). To impose failed dietary models upon people with learning difficulties would be immoral. Therefore all new initiatives should have access to information on successful national practice and 'failed' models in order to achieve effective intervention.

Additionally policy could make some decisions much easier, as seen in the example of food labelling for anyone with poor literacy or numerical skills. The general population are currently grappling with metric weights, so the notion of interpreting numerical nutrition information must be a nightmare. In addition to nutritional labelling complexity, it is time-consuming, and what most people want is surely a simple guide to the possible impact that a product might have on their diet.

Illiteracy is common in our society, so it would seem logical to legislate that food and drink products use simple symbolic food labelling. Symbolic labelling provides a tool for the person with poor literacy skills or sight impairment, as well as the person who prefers to spend time on other pursuits rather than interpreting labels. A symbolic tool could enable people to make wider, more informed choices about their diet. However, the Nutrition Task Force swayed towards meeting the needs of the food and drink industry rather than those of the consumer. It is acknowledged that symbolic food labelling is extremely difficult in terms of meaningful nutrition information, but frameworks could be taken from the food groupings used in the National Plate Model (HEA, 1994). The Food Standards Agency could take the lead and actively pursue the needs of those with poor literacy or numerical skills and sight impairment by demanding that manufacturers change their labelling accordingly. Similarly, other areas where research and policy would support people to make informed choices could be identified.

Access remains a problem in terms of availability, segregation versus inclusion, transport, cost and support. Lifestyle factors, for example exercise, smoking and cervical and breast screening, cannot be addressed unless access to primary health care, health surveillance and health promotion is improved.

Conclusion

People with learning difficulties are currently dependent upon others to make available healthy lifestyle opportunities. In order to change that position, practice, policy, communication and monitoring require consideration.

A national communication network should be established, including user-led groups. Initiatives should be shared and models, particularly those focusing on social inclusion, evaluated. Multi-agency staff training packages and policies supporting the healthy schools/healthy workplaces and healthy neighbourhoods initiatives, as well as HImPs, need to be developed.

Monitoring health outcomes and disease trends among people with learning difficulties is necessary if we are to avoid potentially inaccurate assumptions. While statistics nationally suggest a movement towards the key targets, it is possible that vulnerable groups such as people with learning difficulties are further marginalised. The opportunities are limitless, and with helpful organisational structures in place, people with learning difficulties will enjoy adding life to their years and years to their life.

References

Bendal, E.R.D. and Raybould, E. *The History of the General Nursing Council for England and Wales 1919–1969.* (London: Lewis & Co., 1969).

Carter, G. and Jancar, J. 'Mortality in the mentally handicapped: a fifty year survey at the Stoke Park Group of hospitals (1930–1980)'. *Journal of Mental Deficiency Research,* **27**(1983): 143–56.

Community Care Development Centre. Conference *Towards 2000: The Future Policy for Learning Disability Services.* (London: Kings College, 1997).

Department for Education and Employment. *The Disability Act 1995: What Employers Need to Know.* (London: DfEE, 1996).

Department of Health. *The Health of the Nation: A Consultative Document for Health in England.* (London: HMSO, 1992).

Department of Health. *The Health of the Nation: A Strategy for People with Learning Disabilities.* (Wetherby: DoH, 1995).

Department of Health. *The New NHS, Modern, Dependable.* (London: Stationery Office, 1997a).

Department of Health. *New Health Deal for People with Learning Disabilities* (press release). (London: DoH, 1997b).

Department of Health. *Our Healthier Nation: A Contract for Health: A Consultative Paper.* (London: Stationery Office, 1998a).

Department of Health. *The Healthy Way: How to Stay Healthy – a guide for people with learning disabilities.* (Wetherby: DoH, 1998b).

East Berkshire NHS Trust. Conference *Making Healthier Choices.* (Bracknell: October 1995).

Ewles, L. and Simnett, I. *Promoting Health: A Practical Guide.* (London: Scutari Press, 1995).

Gates, B. 'A new health agenda for learning disabled people: reflections on platitudes and rhetoric.' *Journal of Learning Disabilities for Nursing, Health and Social Care,* **2**(1)(1998): 1–2.

Health Education Authority. *Introducing the National Food Guide: The Balance of Good Health.* (London: HEA, 1994).

Health Education Authority. *Health Related Resources for People with Learning Disabilities.* (London: HEA, 1995).

Hester Adrian Centre for People with Learning Disabilities, conference *The Health of the Nation: Practical Approaches to Healthy Lifestyles.* (University of Manchester, November, 1995).

Howells, G. and Barker, B. 'A protocol for primary health care', in Royal College of General Practitioners *Primary Care for People with a Mental Handicap. Report of a Working Party on the Interface Between the Primary Care Team and People with a Mental Handicap.* RCGP Occasional Paper 47 (London: RCGP, 1990, pp. 12–13).

Lindsey, M. *Signposts for Success in Commissioning and Providing Health Services for People with Learning Disabilities.* (Wetherby: DoH, 1998).

Meehan, S. and Moore, G. 'Specialist services for people with learning disabilities.' *Nursing Times,* **91**(13)(1995): 33–5.

Mencap. *The NHS – Health for all?* (London: Mencap, 1998).

Mental Health Foundation. *Building Expectations: Opportunities and Services for People with a Learning Disability.* Report of the Mental Health Foundation Committee of Inquiry. (1996).

Morton, S. *HIV and People with a Learning Disability.* Paper presented at the East Berkshire NHS Trust Conference. (Bracknell: Mental Health Foundation, October 1995, p. 18).

Naidoo, J. and Wills, J. *Health Promotion: Foundations for Practice.* (London: Baillière Tindall, 1994).

NHS Management Executive. *You Drew a Line and Put Me on One Side of it… Why Should I Suffer?: Learning Disabilities.* (NHSME, 1993).

O'Brien, J. 'A guide to personal planning', in Thomas, G. and Wilcox, B. (eds) *A Comprehensive Guide to the Activities Catalogue: An Alternative for Youth and Adults with Severe Disabilities.* (Baltimore: Paul Brookes, 1987, pp. 1–21).

Rifkin, S.B. and Walt, G. 'Why health improves: defining the issues concerning "comprehensive primary health care" and "selective primary health care".' *Social Science and Medicine,* **6**(1986): 559–66.

Rimmer, J., Braddock D. and Fujiura, G. 'Cardiovascular risk factor levels in adults with mental retardation.' *American Journal on Mental Retardation,* **98**(1994): 510–18.

Rodgers, J. 'Primary health care provision for people with learning difficulties.' *Health and Social Care in the Community,* **2**(1)(1994): 11–17.

St George's Hospital Medical School, Department of Mental Health Sciences. Conference *Enabling People with Learning Disabilities To Use the Health Service.* (London: St George's Hospital Medical School, October 1995).

Simpson, N. *Applying the "Health of the Nation" Policy to People with Learning Disabilities.* Paper presented at conference 'Enabling People with Learning Disabilities To Use the Health Service'. (London: St George's Hospital Medical School, October 1995).

Stein, K. *Primary Care for People with Learning Disabilities: A Survey of Demand, Aspects of Health Service Provision and GP Opinion.* (Southampton Medical School and South West Hants Health Authority, 1996).

Tregelles, J. 'Homelessness: private lives.' *Guardian,* 24 June 1998, p. 8.

Turner, S. and Moss, S. 'The health needs of adults with learning disabilities and the *Health of the Nation* strategy.' *Journal of Intellectual Disability Research,* **40**(1996): 438–50.

2

'ADDING YEARS TO LIFE', BUT ADDING LIFE TO YEARS?

AN INVESTIGATION OF PRIMARY HEALTH CARE

Sid Carter

The chief purpose of primary care is to enhance the health of people by promoting healthy lifestyles and preventing disease. This should be a relatively simple concept, applying to the whole population: surely the notions of health and wellbeing are universally understood by lay people, even if argued about by professionals? Logically, these ideas should remain simple when applied to people with learning difficulties, but various factors combine to make the picture less clear.

This chapter seeks to explore the probable experience of primary health care by a person with a learning difficulty, and some of the practical and ideological issues surrounding this experience. A paradox will be investigated: primary health care is a preoccupation with operationalising 'social justice, equality and individual responsibility for health' (Henk, 1989, p. 12). It has been suggested by writers such as Wolfensberger that the exact reverse of these worthy aims is in fact the main impetus of society towards people with learning difficulties, and indeed for many people with a perceived impairment.

The point is this: primary health care aims to avoid people taking on the mantle of the sick role. How can those with a learning difficulty avoid the sick role when most of the people they meet permanently assign them to it, with or without their permission? The moment that every person who works with people with learning difficulties dreads is that well-meaning eye contact, followed by, 'What's wrong with him, then?' The clear implication is that all impairments not only have a medical origin, but are also patently 'incurable', otherwise someone would have cured them.

Also explored in this chapter is the evidence that people with a learning difficulty do not gain as much from primary care as they could, despite recent improvements in approach. It is suggested that at the root of this lie conflicting approaches, philosophies and ideologies. These prevent positive, consistent moves to enhance the wellbeing of people with learning difficulties.

Overtly and covertly, the world is still debating 'the disability question' in much the same way as the 'Jewish question' was discussed in the 1930s. For example, the mass forced migration of the Jewish people of Europe to Madagascar was a serious suggestion in Nazi circles (Arendt, 1964). The 'Madagascars' for people with learning difficulties are now closing down (at least in their larger form), but witness the recent growth in the call, from varying sources, for care 'villages'. 'What to do with' people with learning difficulties is as yet unresolved in the world, all the options still being open. This ambiguity leads to the largely unsatisfactory delivery of health services to people with learning difficulties. Health means wellbeing, and generally speaking society does not wish people with a learning difficulty well.

Primary health care

Having investigated some of the more accessible UK literature on primary health care, it would be quite possible to gain the impression that it could be defined as essentially anything that occurs in a general practitioner's (GP) surgery. Although this is probably how most people experience it in their daily lives, the notion of primary care is actually more sophisticated than that, being a philosophy to guide the provision of health services world wide.

Although in existence for a long time, primary care gained real momentum from a World Health Organisation (WHO) initiative at Alma Ata in the late 1970s (WHO, 1978). This resulted in the Alma Ata Declaration, committing the signatories (among whom was the UK) to provide health services using the primary care model. This model is founded on the precept of:

> essential health care based on practical, scientifically sound and socially acceptable methods and technology, made universally accessible to individuals and families in the community through their full participation, and at a cost that the community and country can afford to maintain. (WHO, 1978, p. 3)

It can be seen from this statement that the intention of the WHO and supporters of primary care was much more than giving local GPs more responsibility, which is effectively the UK's version of it. In fact, the Alma Ata view of primary health tends to place medical concerns in the wings rather than centre stage. This is demonstrated by the five principles from which the pronouncement quoted above is devolved (WHO, 1978). These are:

1. Equitable distribution
2. Community involvement
3. Appropriate technology
4. A focus on prevention
5. A multisectoral approach.

Factors such as housing, education, nutrition, sanitation and income were seen as having a bigger impact on health than medical interventions, which is echoed in the UK government's blueprint for improving health, *Our Healthier Nation* (DoH, 1998a). Ignoring the political machinations of the international community for the moment, the spirit of the Declaration is obviously worthwhile and is reasonably congruent with the needs of people with learning difficulties. A short analysis of the five principles, related to the needs of people with learning difficulties, demonstrates this.

Equitable distribution is something that would be very welcome for a group of people who have more often than not been denied an ordinary share in resources, health care included.

Community involvement is a theme running through the major ideologies for services for people with learning difficulties: normalisation, social role valorisation.

Appropriate technology is again an important issue. People with learning difficulties have frequently been subject to entirely inappropriate 'technologies' such as corrective neurosurgery and punitive behavioural techniques. Appropriate health technology might be health education, exercise, sport, a balanced diet, physiotherapy, occupational therapy and basic education – but these have often been denied. This is particularly so among the legions of people with learning difficulties who were institutionalised in Europe and the USA.

Focus on prevention is potentially a two-edged sword in terms of a genetic screening interpretation. However, if prevention means, for example, providing high-quality living environments with all the concomitant benefits for the mental and physical wellbeing of a person, this focus is useful.

Multisectoral collaboration. 'Learning difficulties', like any other group label, embraces an enormous range of individuals. At any one time, individuals will have need of different types of help, so having access to a wide range of help can, if well coordinated, only be of value to people with learning difficulties.

Development of, and resistance to, primary health care

Looking at the derivation of the philosophy and practice of primary health provides an instructive insight into the processes of health care delivery. The industrial nations have developed mainly secondary and tertiary health systems, with a resulting technologically advanced, medical and curative approach. This strategy was simply not available to most developing nations as they could not sustain the economic cost. Out of this dilemma grew another way of looking at health. As mentioned before, the major factors in health and wellbeing are non-medical. Also, given sufficient support, these factors can be controlled by local people themselves. Interestingly, this principle has become central to UK health provision, being one of the six key aims that guide the modernisation of the NHS. The Department of Health (DoH) aims:

> To make the delivery of healthcare... a matter of local responsibility. Local doctors and nurses who are in the best position to know what patients need will be in the driving seat in shaping services. (DoH, 1998b, p. 1)

Initiatives based on people's localities started in Africa and Asia as early as the 1920s when community health workers were trained to work in the Sudan (Johnstone and McConnan, 1995). This style of health provision grew rapidly in developing countries, with overall success, leading eventually to the Alma Ata conference in 1977. Despite a universal acceptance of the worthiness of primary care, developed nations mainly supported it through aid programmes to developing countries, while retaining their own traditional systems. Several reasons have been proposed for this reticence. One possible suggestion for this back-pedalling comes from Hall *et al.* (1991), in that nations have found it difficult to identify the most appropriate health professional to take on the role of the primary health worker.

This is despite the suggestion by Dr Halfden Mahler, then Director of the WHO, that nurses are closest to the ideal (Shoultz *et al.*, 1992). This is supported by the inclusion of nurses as an integral part of the primary care groups established by the significant document *The New NHS, Modern, Dependable* (DoH, 1998b).

Another potential reason for the slow uptake of primary care by the West is the power of the medical lobby (Johnstone and McConnan, 1995). The medical infrastructure is very powerful, and primary care undermines the 'top-down' approach of medical science. Allied to this may have been more politics, but on an international level. Many socialist regimes, such as those of China, Cuba and Tanzania, had implemented primary care complete with its concept of local participation and control. Primary care brought great benefits to many of its recipients, as in China, which experienced a tremendous fall in mortality among the under-5s from 1960 onwards, from 175 per 1000 live births to fewer than 49 (World Bank, 1993). Part of the resistance by the West may have been a fear of socialism, and the potential for interpreting the principles of primary care as socialist. Latterly, with the ending of the Cold War and the costs of a curative health system becoming more difficult to bear, Western nations turned their attention to primary care (Shoultz *et al.*, 1992). So, mainly because of economic pressures, the developed nations now also pursue the WHO ideal of Health for All.

Development of primary health care in the UK

Many professional, political, partisan and legislative forces came into play in the late 1980s and 90s to create the health delivery system that we now have in the UK. These are well documented elsewhere, and our attention will now turn to how far the principles of primary health have been followed, and the impact on people with learning difficulties. After all, concurrent with the introduction of a primary health care system into the UK ran the dismantling of large residential facilities for people with learning difficulties. The two projects combined have the potential to make a significant positive impact on the lives of individuals with learning difficulties, that is, providing services that are sensitive to a person's needs and under local control.

In addition, whatever a person's cognitive attributes, so-called individual health behaviour is influenced by social factors. It is approaching either solipsism or extreme behaviourism to suggest that any individual's actions in relation to health can occur totally outside the membership of a social group. This is acknowledged in an influential government publication, *Our Healthier Nation* (DoH, 1998a), which is closer to the principles of Alma Ata. It contains specific references to the social causes of ill health: poverty, unemployment, bad housing and social isolation.

> The Government recognises that the social causes of ill health and the inequalities that stem from them must be acknowledged and acted on. (DoH, 1998a, p. 2)

Prevention and local initiatives are also given more credence. This is certainly encouraging for people with learning difficulties, who experience great social inequality, but problems nevertheless remain.

The impact of primary care on people with learning difficulties

There is a growing body of research on the health needs of people with learning difficulties, from which two main themes emerge. First, people with learning difficulties often have specialist health needs, and second, these are not being met very successfully (RCGP, 1987).

A pioneering piece of research, carried out by Howells (1986), investigated the health needs of 151 adults with learning difficulties attending a day care centre. Many easily treated health problems came to light, mainly unknown to the person's GP. In the group were 34 people with Down's syndrome, only two of whom had been tested for hypothyroidism, a common disorder in people with this syndrome. Eight out of the 151 individuals had undiagnosed hypertension, while 20 people were significantly overweight. Help with weight reduction had not been offered. Only three of the 13 people with epilepsy were given regular reviews to determine the effectiveness of their treatment. Howells found further undiagnosed or ignored health problems: scabies, head lice, and various conditions that impaired the vision or hearing of individuals. He suggested various reasons why such apparently routine and easily avoided health difficulties might have occurred:

1. GPs may assume that responsibility lies with specialists rather than with themselves.

2. Individuals under-report their symptoms for various reasons, for example, communication difficulties or a belief that discomfort must simply be borne.
3. The individual may not find that the standard surgery system suits their (or their carer's) requirements, and may thus not attend.

Cole (1986) conducted a similar study in another day care service, investigating the health needs of 53 adults. Out of this group, 35 people had unattended health needs, and four individuals needed help urgently. Only 15 had been to see their GP since leaving school. These findings were echoed by Wilson and Haire (1990), who examined 65 adults with a learning difficulty on simple health parameters such as vision and hearing. They found that 57 of these people had a detectable health need, and the authors expressed concern that 26 individuals were receiving repeat prescriptions of anticonvulsant or psychiatric drugs without regular review.

An Australian study found undiagnosed health needs in 66 per cent of the 251 people with learning difficulties studied (Beange and Bauman, 1990). The proposition that people with learning difficulties receive inadequate primary health care compared with the general population is further supported by a study in the South-West of England. Langan *et al.* (1993) used the more rigorous methodology of matched controls when investigating the health care delivered to 90 adults with learning difficulties. This research found that the control group received preventive health interventions more frequently than did the group of people with learning difficulties. Birenbaum (1995) suggests that present trends in the way in which public health services are managed in the USA mean that people with learning difficulties will be competing for increasingly scarce primary health care resources.

A study carried out in the UK also examined the issue of resources in primary health care for people who have learning difficulties. Stein (1996) surveyed 48 GPs as a result of concerns about the adequacy of services following the closure of an institution for people with learning difficulties. He also undertook a case note review of 112 people and investigated the uptake of breast and cervical screening. Stein found that the respondents reported more consultations than average among their patients with learning difficulties, but that they were too small in number to justify very much extra training. Most of the GPs had little contact with specialist teams. The uptake of breast and cervical screening was considerably less than in the general population. One of the most interesting aspects of this study lies in its methodology, particularly when set in the context of the empowerment ideology of primary health care:

It was decided not to involve people with a learning disability or their carers directly in the survey [as this] would be more time consuming. (Stein, 1996, p. 10)

These studies provide strong evidence of the poor quality of primary health care received by most people with learning difficulties, but also convey the relative ease of increasing quality dramatically. The key factor appears to be an awareness that people with learning difficulties may need extra help to achieve optimum health. This help could be in the form of a change in professional attitudes, for example an acceptance that people with learning difficulties are sexual beings and thus have the same sexual health needs as everyone else. If this were the case, better access to sex education, contraceptive advice, cervical screening and similar health interventions might well follow. Extra help could also be delivered as increased professional skills, such as more diligent listening to people with learning difficulties, more creative ways of testing vision and hearing, and so on.

This has to some extent been recognised in the extensive guidelines for commissioning and providing health services for people with learning difficulties, *Signposts for Success* (Lindsey, 1998). In this advisory document, the DoH presents a comprehensive account, based on wide consultation, of how people with learning difficulties should benefit from the NHS.

Positive primary health care for people with learning difficulties

Despite the impression that government proclamations appear to lack real power, there is encouraging evidence that people with learning difficulties do not, by definition, have to endure substandard primary health care. Additionally, better care does not necessarily mean a huge additional demand on resources. Innovative practice has been reported that endeavours to solve some of the problems highlighted above, and importantly, at no great extra cost.

As mentioned, the obstacles to providing comprehensive primary health care to people with learning difficulties in the USA are potentially enormous. Despite this, a service has been established in New Jersey that works within existing funding arrangements and has made a significant impact on the health of the people with learning difficulties that it serves (Criscione *et al.*, 1994). The facility is a developmental disabilities centre based at a hospital in the New Jersey area. Initially, most of the work was carried out at the centre itself, but its work has increasingly become consultative. This both widens the area of influence and helps to promote community integration. One of the major problems reported in providing primary health care to people with learning difficulties is that any particular professional will only see a relatively small number of individuals with a learning difficulty. This makes it unlikely that he or she will gain any real expertise. The initiative in New Jersey counteracts this by bringing together professionals who do have the necessary expertise, making this available to primary care workers who need it. If necessary, people attend the centre itself, but wherever possible they remain in their own localities, seeing their local primary care professional. The centre provides support to community-based primary care workers who are interested in helping people with learning difficulties, training and collaboration with various community integration programmes.

Important though these activities are, the authors claim that the real difference is made by the 'health coordination' activities of the centre's nurse practitioners. This health coordination basically consists of making sure that interventions are made to promote healthy lifestyles and to prevent, or at least detect, disease. This includes mental health, environmental and behavioural aspects of health.

The centre actively supports research and evaluation, and these have demonstrated significant health gains, by promoting positive health and by the early detection of health needs that would otherwise have gone unnoticed. When people did need hospital services, their stays were shorter and more successful, that is, less likely to lead to readmission. This alone meant financial savings, which has already been proposed as one of the main reasons why governments have adopted the primary health care model.

Another example of good practice in providing good-quality primary health care is described by Meehan *et al.* (1995). Meehan and her colleagues established a well person clinic at a day service, having found through a pilot study a series of undiagnosed health needs. This was not intended to replace existing primary care services, but simply to provide a user-friendly introduction to health promotion and screening. Simple but thorough investigations were carried out with 191 adults with a learning difficulty, discovering 176 people with undetected but easily treatable conditions, many with more than one. All the findings were within the parameters of an ordinary GP's sphere of investigations. This innovative practice did not use any special technology or expensive techniques. Put simply, the technology used was a way of thinking; people with learning difficulties have health needs in the same way as the general population do.

In the late 1980s, the Royal College of General Practitioners (RCGP) initiated a working party on how best to accommodate people with learning difficulties in primary care, which led to the publication of a report (RCGP, 1987). This was a heartening move, the report consisting of a series of papers on how GPs might deal with a selection of situations, epilepsy and Down's syndrome among them. The information for each topic is relatively brief, but the list of recommendations is long and wide ranging. Thus, although the report is essentially a positive step, it at the same time illustrates the problems involved in providing primary health care in a medically dominated system.

This is further illustrated by the results of a questionnaire sent to Greenwich GPs (Holt, 1992). Less than a quarter of respondents had referred a patient to the community learning disability team. Eighty per cent wanted further information about what services were provided. This indicates that perhaps many GPs simply do not have enough information to offer good-quality primary health care to those of their patients who have learning difficulties.

The barriers facing GPs when dealing with people who have learning difficulties are eloquently described by Howells (1995). He describes the prejudice and misinformation surrounding learning difficulties that exist in the medical profession. However, he also demonstrates how a simple change of attitude can revolutionise a GP's practice. Despite being far from ideal, the UK's medically dominated version of primary health care could meet the health needs of people with learning difficulties, provided that GPs were well informed and well trained.

The successes described above by Meehan *et al.* and Criscione *et al.* were totally congruent with *Our Healthier Nation*-type principles and targets, but were only achieved by side stepping existing primary care systems. The systems established to achieve good health had failed these particular individuals with learning difficulties, and it is safe to assume that they fail many more. An important factor to note is that both schemes were rooted in actively valuing people with learning difficulties. This is in stark contrast to the more prevalent tolerance or energetic devaluing of people with learning difficulties.

Health care in a devaluing society

We return here to the incongruity mentioned at the beginning of this chapter, that is, that the mainly indifferent primary care provided to people with learning difficulties is the result of society's lack of clarity about how to treat this group of people. Put baldly, what is the purpose of improving the health of a person whose very existence is in question? The ambivalence of the public towards people with learning difficulties is demonstrated by comparing the coverage of two issues, the quality of life of Thomas Creedon, a boy with learning difficulties, and genetic engineering of the non-disabled population, both of which have received media attention.

Thomas Creedon, who in the summer of 1995 was 22 months old, was reported to have brain damage and no sight or hearing, and to cry inconsolably most of the time. His parents claimed that Thomas had a very poor quality of life, and thus believed that the artificial feeding he received through a tube in his stomach should cease. This issue has become the subject of a court case. Shamash (1995, p. 14) wrote that doctors and nurses 'face dilemmas in ethics, as improved methods of treatment make it possible to extend lives, which, some would consider, are scarcely worth preserving'. These are the same health professionals who are exhorted to uphold the lofty ideals of Health for All. It is no wonder that primary health care for most people who have learning difficulties is an uneasy compromise.

Contrast Thomas Creedon's media portrayal, most of which echoed the sentiments above, with that of the debate over genetic engineering. Suggestions that science should intervene to reduce differences in humans other than those perceived as disabilities are met with a public outcry. The idea of scientists being able to change the genetic material of 'normal' fetuses to alter height, gender, eye colour and similar parameters produces widespread unease. This is demonstrated by Appleyard's (1996) discussion of how odd he felt in supporting the resistance of the deaf community to any supposed 'cure' for deafness. Lewis Wolpert, a supporter of genetic engineering, talks about the rigorous safeguards imposed on genetic scientists to stop them working on anything other than 'preventable disease' (Wolpert, 1996). The value and integrity of a person without impairment approaches absolute, but a person with, or destined to have, an impairment can legitimately be seen as worthless. In the hierarchy of such impairments, learning difficulties is in a prominent position, as evidenced by the prevalence of testing to prevent Down's syndrome.

A comparison of Thomas Creedon and genetic engineering does not itself mean that the argument is cut and dried. However, it illustrates the difference in public perception once the factor of learning difficulties is introduced. Health professionals are also members of society, so are influenced by these perceptions.

Conclusion

This chapter has sought to demonstrate that primary health care for people with learning difficulties in the UK is deeply flawed, for two main reasons. First, the medicalised, GP-led version of primary care practised in the UK is unsuited to a lot of people with learning difficulties (Cook, 1998). Evidence suggests that despite being more congruent with the liberating Health for All principle, the new primary care-led NHS will be dominated by doctors (North *et al.*, 1998). Second, the attitudes of many people towards their fellow citizens who have learning difficulties contain a subtext, namely that they would be better off dead.

To counteract these difficulties, evidence has been presented that good-quality primary health care for people with learning difficulties is possible given important changes. Most importantly, the lives of people with learning difficulties need to be positively valued. Meehan *et al.*'s well person clinic demonstrates the power of this essential attitude shift. It is within the capacity of any health professional to effect this change, and this would result in a major improvement in health care. Also, if the UK completely adopted the non-medical, localised version of primary health care that has evolved in developing nations, people with learning difficulties would have a greater chance of being participants in their own health.

People with learning difficulties are undoubtedly living longer and having years added to life. Research shows that it is relatively straightforward to offer good-quality primary health care to people, even if their needs are fairly specialised. Thus, if health professionals are aware of this and value service users who have learning difficulties, they will be on the right road to adding life to years.

Checklist for action

- Health professionals should have valuing attitudes. For real progress to be made, it should be clear policy in the health services that the lives of people with learning difficulties have a value equal to those of everybody else. People with learning difficulties need unequivocal human rights.
- Primary health care should be conceived of as citizens being helped to take control of their own health needs.
- Primary health care as practised in the UK is strongly medically led, bureaucratic and hierarchical. This should be changed in line with the proposals of *Our Healthier Nation* (DoH, 1998a) in order to reflect the original empowering version of primary health care, which better suits the needs of people with learning difficulties.
- Health professionals need to be well prepared and have access to specialist help when needed, so that people with learning difficulties can enjoy positive health care.

References

Appleyard, B. 'There's more to life than being Joe Normal: as medical technology allows us to avoid "abnormality", we risk seeing difference as illness.' *The Independent*, 6 June 1996.

Arendt, H. *Eichmann in Jerusalem: A Report on the Banality of Evil* (2nd edn). (Harmondsworth: Penguin, 1964).

Beange, H. and Bauman, A. 'Health care for the developmentally disabled. Is it necessary?', in Fraser W. (ed.) *Key Issues in Mental Retardation Research*. (London: Routledge, 1990, p. 154–62).

Birenbaum, A. 'Managed care and the future of primary care for adults with mental retardation.' *Mental Retardation*, **33**(5)(1995): 334–7.

Cole, O. 'Medical screening of adults at social education centres: whose responsibility?', *Mental Handicap*, **14**(6)(1986): 54–6.

Cook, H. 'Primary health care for people with learning disabilities.' *Nursing Times*, **94**(30)(1998): 54–5.

Criscione, T., Kastner, T.A., O'Brien, D. and Nathanson, R. 'Replication of a managed health care initiative for people with mental retardation living in the community.' *Mental Retardation*, **32**(1)(1994): 43–52.

Department of Health. *Our Healthier Nation*. (London: Stationery Office, 1998a).

Department of Health. *The New NHS, Modern, Dependable*. (London: Stationery Office, 1998b).

Hall, J., Ross, A.S., Edge, D. and Pynn, G.A. 'Primary health care – a nursing model: a Danish–Newfoundland (Canada) project', in Norton, P.G., Stewart, M., Tudiver, F., Bass, M.J. and Dunn, E.V. (eds) *Primary Care Research*. (London: Sage, 1991, p. 195–208).

Henk, M.L. (ed.) *Social Work in Primary Care*. (Newbury Park, CA: Sage, 1989).

Holt, G. 'Primary care for people with mental handicaps.' *Psychiatric Bulletin*, **16**(10)(1992): 667.

Howells, G. 'Are the medical needs of mentally handicapped adults being met?' *Journal of the Royal College of General Practitioners*, **36**(1986): 449–56.

Howells, G. *Primary Medical Care for People with Learning Disability: Overcoming the Barriers*. Paper presented at conference 'Enabling People with Learning Disabilities To Use the Health Service'. (London: St Georges Hospital Medical School, 1995).

Johnstone, P.A. and McConnan, I. 'Primary health care led NHS learning from developing countries.' *British Medical Journal*, **311**(7010)(1995): 891–2.

Langan, J., Russell, O. and Whitfield, M. Community Care and the General Practitioner. Primary Health Care for People with Learning Disabilities. Unpublished report to the Department of Health. (Bristol: Norah Fry Research Centre, 1993).

Lindsey, M. *Signposts for Success in Commissioning and Providing Health Services for People with Learning Disabilities*. (London: DoH, 1998).

Meehan, S., Moore, G. and Barr, O. 'Specialist services for people with learning disabilities.' *Nursing Times*, **91**(13)(1995): 33–5.

North, N., Lupton, C., Khan, P. and Lacey, D. 'Altogether now: *The New NHS* White Paper.' *Nursing Times*, **94**(33)(1998): 38–40.

Royal College of General Practitioners. *Primary Care for People with a Mental Handicap. Report of a Working Party on the Interface between the Primary Care Team and People with a Mental Handicap*. (London: RCGP, 1987).

Shamash, J. 'Measures for comfort and joy.' *Nursing Times*, **91**(33)(1995): 14–15.

Shoultz, J., Hatcher, P.A. and Hurrell, M. 'Growing edges of a new paradigm: the future of nursing in the health of the nation.' *Nursing Outlook*, **40**(2)(1992): 57–61.

Stein, K. *Primary Care for People with Learning Disability: A Survey of Demand, Aspects of Health Service Provision and GP Opinion*. (Southampton: Southampton and South West Hants Health Authority, 1996).

Wilson, N. and Haire, A. 'Health care screening for people with a mental handicap living in the community.' *British Medical Journal*, **301**(1990): 1379–81.

Wolpert, L. 'Science: hypotheses.' *The Independent on Sunday*, 12 May 1996.

World Bank. *World Development Report* (Oxford: World Bank, 1993).

World Health Organisation. *Primary Health Care. Report of the International Conference on Primary Health Care*. (Geneva: WHO, 1978).

3

A MODEL FOR PROGRAMMES PROMOTING HEALTHY LIFESTYLES

Roberta Astor and Karen Jeffereys

Our Healthier Nation (DoH, 1998) emphasised the impact that lifestyle has upon health. While acknowledging that 'Life is by its nature risky' (DoH, 1998, p. 34), it is agreed that people need to know about risks to health in order to make informed judgements about how to avoid or minimise those risks. Greenhalgh observes that for people with learning difficulties, 'little or no work so far has looked at their needs for information about health issues' (DMHS, 1995, p. 31).

This chapter describes the authors' experiences in running health promotion programmes as a way of enabling healthy choices for people with learning difficulties. The programmes were based upon the Health Education Authority (HEA) Look After Yourself (LAY) model, now superseded by contextualised National Vocational Qualification training.

Using HEA-advocated structure and information ensures the correct use of contemporary, evidence-based information for health promotion. There is, however, a lack of information or guidelines available for running health promotion programmes with people who have severe learning difficulties and/or multiple disabilities. By sharing the mistakes and successes experienced when running these programmes, it is hoped that issues will be raised and ideas for health promotion development in this area encouraged. The ideas described could be used by staff providing learning disability services with the caveat that practitioners should ensure that health promotion is based on contemporary, accurate evidence.

The aim of the LAY programme was 'to offer a systematic programme leading to learning opportunities which enable the individual to develop knowledge, motivation and skills in order that he/she can optimise the physical and psychological determinants of his/her own health' (HEA, 1994a, p. 5). More specifically LAY was about (HEA, 1994a, p. 7):

- Positive lifestyle, rather than the management of disease.
- Enabling individuals to achieve what is appropriate for them by starting from where they are in terms of their perceptions, values, and priorities.
- Focusing on the encouragement of independent skills which will enable individuals to make health-promoting decisions for the rest of their lives. Underpinning this is the development of their self-esteem, confidence and ability to control/influence their situation.

Programmes using this approach allow individual skill and knowledge development in a group setting by focusing upon both health improvement and the reduction of health risk factors, within an enjoyable social environment. Competence gained in this way needs to be integrated into a person's lifestyle to prevent the programmes becoming isolated health education and therefore unlikely to truly promote health. It is not helpful to push lifestyle change aims at a group of people who may have little or no control over their lives.

Health promotion for people with learning difficulties should use adult learning methodology, empowering people to make informed choices and take control over their own health.

Programme structure

The programmes described here were divided into three components: physical activity/exercise, relaxation and various health topics. Each component specifically selected was the safest method for people who have little or no knowledge or skills in that particular area. The aim is that over the period of a 6–10-week course, individuals work at their own pace and level, gradually building on their own skills. Competitiveness is discouraged; thus a more skilled person, for example someone who regularly exercises, will be encouraged to work at his or her own level without it affecting others' self-esteem. Additionally, an opt-out clause should enable all participants to opt out of a particular activity if they so wish.

General points to consider

Venue, access, safety and cost require consideration when planning programmes. The ideal venue would be a local community leisure/sports centre. Unfortunately, cost often precludes the use of such a place. 'Healthy living centres' could provide space for programmes in which all local people could participate. This would promote social inclusion and 'healthy neighbourhoods'.

Venues need to be free if possible and within easy travelling distance. A large room is needed for exercise and relaxation, one in which noise can be made without disturbing the building's other occupants. Wheelchair access may be needed. Toilets and facilities to make drinks are necessary, and somewhere to store equipment is a hoped-for luxury.

It is useful to buy beverages in bulk and ask a small weekly charge to cover cost. An initial 'getting to know you' session is crucial and can include issues concerned with group confidentiality and group ground rules.

Participants should wear loose, comfortable clothing and appropriate footwear.

Medical information should be acquired prior to a person starting the programme and is normally included in a preliminary questionnaire. Further information and possibly medical assurance on the safety of the person participating can subsequently be sought.

Insurance liability for programme facilitators needs consideration. Their employer's indemnity insurance cover might apply, but it should be ascertained how this works should a programme participant decide to sue a programme facilitator as an individual. Programme facilitators will be responsible for the health and safety of their groups, and should take precautions for accident prevention, as well as steps to ensure safe action in the event of fire or accidents.

Description of programmes run by the authors

The authors ran seven health promotion programmes in total, facilitating two together. For the rest, they teamed up with other people, some of whom were training as LAY tutors, for example an occupational therapist, a Mencap Homes Foundation manager, a dental health educator and a non LAY-trained community nurse. Programme participants were clients or staff from the health, social or non-statutory services. No participating staff held relevant professional qualifications. Each programme had between eight and 16 participants.

The description of the programmes will consider the intentions behind attempting a partnership approach between staff and clients. Mistakes, successes and participant response during the programmes will be recounted using LAY components as a structure. All the programmes discussed offered all three components – exercise, relaxation and a health topic – from the beginning, emphasising each equally.

A partnership approach, with mutual support between clients and staff, was an aim for five programmes. It was hoped that people would help each other to learn and share their individual strengths and weaknesses. All the clients required one-to-one support, especially during the early stages; a staff partner would give a familiar, consistent approach. There were particular needs among non-verbal clients as none had been enabled to use symbols or sign language as an effective means of communication. One client had learnt Makaton at school, but a lack of support in using the skill at home precluded the use of Makaton during the programme. Attendance on the programme by a staff member from this person's home would have made this possible as both the client and the staff member could have learnt Makaton relevant to the expression of a healthy lifestyle choice and action during the programme and extended this to the home environment.

Partnerships between clients and staff would enable the practice of exercise and relaxation at home, plus an expansion of other health gain activities. A broad aim was for people to achieve a level whereby they could safely use community facilities for health gain. This needed staff to recognise and advocate for any necessary environmental changes. In short, attempting a partnership approach aimed for 'clients and workers collaborating to promote positive wellbeing and informed choice' (Greenhalgh, 1994, p. 14). The degree to which this was achieved will be detailed during description of programmes.

Exercise

On most programmes, at least half an hour a week was devoted to exercise. The start of each programme provided a complementary health topic based on the benefits of exercise. Emphasis was placed on establishing a personal exercise programme. This was to consist first of flexibility exercises, aimed at increasing and retaining joint mobility, to be performed at least three times a week. These provided a useful 'warm up' before the demand of other types of exercise. Current HEA advice is that pulse raising activities that gradually increase in intensity should precede stretching exercises to reduce the risk to cold muscles, all forming part of the 'warm up'.

Second, 15–60 minutes of continuous or discontinuous aerobic activity to promote cardiovascular health to be performed three to five times a week, followed by a gradual pulse lowering activity.

Third, muscular strength and endurance exercises to be performed two to three times per week in order to promote the safe ability to perform some everyday activities, to maintain good posture and to help to avoid back pain. It was not viewed as problematic if people did not always include muscular strength and endurance exercises in their regime.

Although individuals could work at their own pace and level of ability, the programme ethos encouraged everyone to attempt everything. However, an opt-out clause was allowed, particularly when a specific exercise was contraindicated for health reasons. It is important to recognise that the majority of participants may be unfit or new to being more active, and therefore need time before handling cardiovascular exercise. In addition, the whole regime may not be appropriate for everyone, although a balanced exercise programme should be achieved. The 3-year Active for Life Campaign, launched by the HEA in March 1996, promotes 30 minutes' physical activity most days of the week.

Monitoring progress

LAY advocated monitoring progress by the 'talk test' – being able to talk throughout exercise – the rate of perceived exertion (RPE), pulse counting and personal exercise records. Initially, both pulse count and RPE should be recorded to examine their relationship. The 'talk test' proved the only method that truly worked for participants with a learning difficulty. Even this, however, proved problematic for non-verbal people. A close watch was kept for signs of overexertion during exercise.

The use of pulse counting, RPE and personal exercise records was attempted. Much time was wasted taking pulses for people and trying to teach them to do so themselves. Neither clients nor staff ever managed to use pulse counting for monitoring. Some people pretended by holding their wrists and saying any number that sounded right to them. RPE could not be related to pulse counting so it was used to help people to relate how they felt to their level of exercise performance.

Personal exercise records were useless. LAY-issue record cards, with tiny tick boxes, were modified by an occupation therapist LAY tutor, using pictures and colour coordination. Clients wanted to use these but could not complete them unaided. On programmes where staff dropped out, clients asked programme facilitators to complete the records or wrote their made-up number somewhere on the chart. No records were completed to monitor home exercise. Record cards designed to meet the needs of this client group would be useful. Thought should also be given to designing an RPE scale using symbols or signs and taking into account the needs of people with visual disabilities.

Aids for pulse taking are available. For one programme, the local health promotion unit lent one that clipped on like an earring. This worked well and people wanted to use it, but only one was available and then only on one occasion.

For the first programme, the HEA provided a fitness monitoring bicycle and a member of staff to help people to use it. A mini 'physical' checked participants' blood pressures and pulses. This proved popular, and it was hoped that a repeat session at the end of the programme would measure achievement. Unfortunately, the bicycle when provided without support was too complicated to operate.

In some cases, all the relevant medical information had not been disclosed on the preliminary questionnaire. One woman's pulse rate did not rise above 60 beats per minute after bicycle use. Questioning discovered that she took beta blockers, not indicated on her form. She was asked to give a letter explaining the programme to her doctor to gain his advice, he expressed delight at her participation. Consequently, it was insisted that forms be returned to programme facilitators before programme commencement, people being referred to their doctors if there was any doubt. However, a non-disclosure of relevant health status details still occurred. This raises issues about access to the correct health details for clients and their staff.

Exercise programme

During the first programme, clients remained committed. Unfortunately, the number of staff rapidly dwindled to one person attending regularly and a few others intermittently. Teaching and monitoring exercise was hectic. At the time, LAY recommended teaching a sequence of movements for suppleness and strength performed at different levels according to ability. All the movements needed accuracy for benefit and safety. One client with a short concentration span would only perform movements once or twice, next to a programme facilitator, before running off. Other clients would only do the movements if given one-to-one attention. The movements were too complicated for any clients to achieve much independence.

The participant taking beta blockers was very energetic and could compete during exercise. A fellow participant would only run holding one end of a skipping rope while being led by someone holding the other. Teaming these two succeeded in maintaining a pace beneficial to both. It was acknowledged that two people running while holding skipping rope ends looks strange, so chasing the person in front was encouraged as a replacement strategy.

One man opted out of cardiovascular exercise. He remained behind when the group ran, promising to walk briskly. He probably had a rest instead, but he was not pressurised or criticised for this choice.

Everyone exercised during this programme, but real success was achieved only for a person who started using local leisure and sports facilities. She also bought a treadmill and uses it regularly, also still visiting the local gym. As she is young and perceived as restless, this is an excellent energy channel.

For another programme, the authors borrowed an exercise bicycle and rowing machine. Skipping ropes, hula hoops and a large, soft ball were also used to motivate reluctant exercisers, making activity fun. Committed attendance by both clients and staff made exercise sessions easier to run. One staff participant, a marathon runner, took some of the group on a regular short run. The client participant for whom this man was a staff member found running easy and enjoyable, which led to a shared interest outside the programme.

One woman only reluctantly exercised for moments before retreating. On the last session, she came forward and started belly dancing. Her staff member said that she had attended dancing classes. The authors realised that they had focused too narrowly when discussing the benefits of exercise and exploring activity levels. Sports, forms of brisk exercise and disco dancing had been related to cardiovascular benefit. If raising activity levels generally had been advocated, this woman could have belly danced during the exercise component and probably interested others.

Another participant had severe, multiple disabilities. A passive exercise programme was devised that she could practise to music at home with the help of staff. The movements were videotaped to aid home use. The movements only increased suppleness and were approved by a physiotherapist. If asked, a physiotherapist could have recommended movements that gave cardiovascular benefit, but this was not realised at the time.

Pleasant, slow music was incorporated for everyone's suppleness exercises, and lively music was sometimes used to motivate cardio-vascular exercise. It should be ensured that exercise is with and not to music.

On one programme, participants were clients and staff from Mencap residences. The author involved perceived the clients as being very able, even though they were described as having severe learning difficulties. The discussion of the benefits of exercise consid-ered everyday activity as well as sport. Consequently, programme participants started to garden and take long walks to improve their fitness, recognising the benefits of different activity levels.

The venue for this programme was a small room in a building situated in a busy town high street. All exercise had to take place in the room. Cardiovascular exercise was difficult. Music successfully promoted all the exercises once people had gained competence. The clients' high level of ability and the excellent staff support enabled everyone to learn all the complicated movements to a reasonable standard.

Space and facilities will always dictate the types of physical activity. On one course, run on church premises, a large sports hall was used. Although it was somewhat large for group discussion, it provided excellent opportunities for a variety of energetic activities. Circuit training, ball games, skipping and running were included. Additionally, one woman who used a wheelchair was able to develop and practise the skill of throwing a soft ball into a basket-ball net. Her pleasure at successfully participating in team games such as these was shared by the whole group.

In some situations, it might be felt that there is not enough space to carry out physical activity; in two courses, run with a learning disability community nurse, this was certainly the case. However, rather than omit this component, armchair exercises to music were used. Music from popular television 'soap opera' programmes was used, proving to be an extremely motivating and enjoyable addi-tion. It was hoped that by using soap opera theme music, people would be motivated to move, even for 1 minute, when watching these programmes at home, thus building activity into their regular daily lifestyle. Participants were also encouraged to lead the activity instead of the facilitators doing so; this empowered people and increased their confidence. On one programme, one man became particularly good at leading the group, then wishing to share his skills with other people using the day services that he attended. This was discussed with his key worker but was unfortunately never taken further because of a lack of support from within the service. This was without doubt an opportunity lost for many of the day service consumers, and particularly for the man himself.

Relaxation

Relaxation is known to be integral to people's wellbeing, and people with learning difficulties are certainly being given the opportunity to experience relaxation sessions. Specifically, LAY used a neuro-muscular tension control relaxation programme (HEA, 1994a, p. 127–39), a model based upon the work of Joe Macdonald Wallace, who developed work of Edmund Jacobson. This is difficult for many people with learning difficulties and requires the tutor to demon-strate clearly the action required in each relaxation session.

In the authors' experience, a more appropriate approach is to select parts of this core relaxation programme and combine them with parts of the relaxation extension module. This relaxation extension module focuses upon overall body awareness and balance rather than tension awareness in a specific muscle group. People are encouraged to try different positions in order to find their own optimum comfort. Many people find lying down uncom-fortable, so encouraging them to explore various sitting positions is helpful. On some of the courses, the space available or a cold floor limited people's positions. Again, when space was at a premium, armchair relaxation was focused upon. In some venues, mats were available; in others, people had to bring their own blankets. Where floor space was available, a technique known as 'placing out' (extension module), taken from massage therapies, was used to help people physically to experience their body lying in a position conducive to relaxation.

Each person requires individual attention to ensure that he or she is gaining the most from the session. Some people prefer to keep their eyes open in the initial stages. On one course, a woman with severe physical and learning difficulties benefited by having aromatherapy and foot massage during the session, and this was continued by the staff at home. On another course, one woman found it very difficult to remain still and quiet, initially interrupting the sessions for other participants. Over the weeks, however, people found her movements less invasive, and she also found a more comfortable and acceptable position on a beanbag. In addition, one very active member of staff found it extremely difficult to learn the skills of relaxation. Conversely, some people found this extremely easy and often fell asleep.

Feedback from this session relies upon the tutors' observation of each individual in all stages of relaxation, particularly those who are unable to feedback their experiences verbally. Carefully selected music, although not advocated in the LAY relaxation programme, was used in some courses, usually in their latter parts. In these situations when people had experienced relaxation with and without music, they chose to have quiet background music. Some people took their own audiotape with a view to practising at home. Overall, this component of the programme was looked forward to, people generally enjoying the relaxation. However, few people actually practised at home.

Health topics

For the first programme, the topics were imposed, but on subsequent programmes, the participants were asked to choose them. The decision to allow choice came from the painful experience of trying to explain coronary heart disease as a topic on the first programme. Staff were interested but clients switched off. The authors decided that a discussion based on an understanding of health and its affecting factors would be more appropriate. This discussion determined the subsequent programme content.

With experience, it was learnt that people wanted to address a number of different topics, including sleep, back care and the signs and symptoms of being unwell. This section describes each health topic, the approaches used and anecdotal successes and failures.

Coronary heart disease

For the Mencap programme, large, colourful diagrams of the heart and a piece of pipe stuffed with foam rubber were used to demonstrate physiological mechanisms. Participants shared their knowledge of heart disease and risk factors by relating to people whom they knew who had suffered from angina or a heart attack. This worked well because of the participants' high level of ability. One woman had a history of deep vein thrombosis; she was also overweight and smoked. The session content initially frightened her. She thought that it meant she would have a heart attack and because she smoked, people would blame her. The group reassured her that they did not blame her. She was told that the risk factors for coronary heart disease did not mean that she was going to die but that she had control. She cheered up with encouraging attention from the group to make healthy lifestyle choices. On many courses, coronary heart disease was not focused upon as a topic. It was felt that people needed the skills to prevent coronary heart disease rather than just knowledge.

Healthy eating

An approach to healthy eating was taken by looking at the whole diet in terms of what, why and how to make changes, the aim being to reach the targets of eating less fat and sugar, and more fruit, vegetables and starchy foods. The food group system (HEA, 1994b, p. 149) pre-empted the National Plate Model (the Balance of Good Health) produced by the Nutrition Task Force, which was a working group for *The Health of the Nation* strategy (HEA, 1994b). Although an excellent model, this has problems for a person with learning difficulties because it relies upon people's knowledge of basic foods. Through the professional experience of one of the authors, it was known that programmes needed to focus on one particular aspect rather than on generalised statements about diet. On some programmes, people were so interested in the topic that two sessions were included. Sessions covered three key areas: reducing fat, increasing fruit and vegetables, and reducing sugar in the diet. The most successful sessions included real food and vivid visual cues.

Fruit and vegetables often formed the major focus of a session. Brainstorming on available fresh, frozen, dried or tinned produce provides a baseline of people's knowledge. This can be followed by tasting a range of fruit and vegetables, including new or exotic varieties. Making this a social event inspires a natural discussion on people's likes, dislikes and habits and it becomes easy to encourage them to eat more fruit and vegetables. On one programme, a woman revealed that she was not allowed to eat a lot of fruit

43

because of a bowel problem. Later investigation revealed that the woman had been treated for bowel cancer but was unaware of her diagnosis as relatives had not wanted her to know.

Sugar in the diet was focused upon by vividly demonstrating the quantities of sugar, in teaspoons, in a range of food and drink. This time-tested method continues to shock some people and forms the basis for quizzes ('guess the number of teaspoons in...') and debate.

Blindfold tasting can help people to overcome prejudices about certain foods. The opt-out clause must obviously be exercised with this type of activity as some would find this too frightening. However, tasting wholemeal versus white bread, and low-fat spread versus butter, met with the approval of the programme participants. Taste, current eating habits and health benefits can be discussed.

Two methods that addressed the whole diet were tried out. One was to produce meals on paper plates using pictures from magazines and discussing the health benefits or risk factors. The other used jigsaws made from food photographs in the shape of a 'healthy' heart and a 'broken' heart.

For one programme food diaries, and for another fruit and vegetable diaries, were attempted in order to help people to recall their usual eating habits. Neither was particularly helpful as people either forgot to return them or had no support outside the programme to complete them.

It is unfortunate that symbolic nutrition labelling does not exist as it would provide an ideal tool for people easily to identify the health gains from particular foods.

To complement the healthy eating topic, a wide range of drinks was available throughout most programmes. Choices included water, ordinary and decaffeinated coffee and tea, herbal teas, low-sugar squashes and fruit juices. Sweeteners, sugar and low-fat milks were used. People were encouraged to try new drinks.

Smoking

The Mencap programme looked at how to support people to stop smoking. Only one participant smoked and she wanted to cut down. Other participants showed concern for friends or relatives who smoked and about the effects of passive smoking. HEA leaflets offering advice were eagerly taken home, although only one client could read.

This topic was often not chosen by participants on other programmes because few people smoked. However, on some, the effects of 'passive' smoking were discussed. Additionally, people identified places where others smoked, 'no smoking' signs and the use of no smoking areas in social and residential settings. People were encouraged to recognise their rights and the control of their own health by moving away, using no smoking areas and possibly asking people not to smoke in their home or work environments.

Uses and abuses of drugs

This topic considered prescription drugs and those purchased over the counter. Participants were asked for a list of drugs they took and kept in their bathroom cabinets. The aim was to raise the awareness about medication generally, the reasons for taking it, its correct use and storage and alternatives to drug taking. A jar full of pill-like sweets and medicine cups with measures of juice aided discussion. Participants were given juice or a sweet and asked, 'If that is parac-etamol (or any drug example from their lists), will you swallow it?' This enabled people to say when and whether they would take the drug without revealing their personal list contents. Many non-verbal participants smiled or shook their heads in response to infor-mation given about the drug by their group. Mencap programme participants refused the sweet reward because the healthy eating component of the course had warned them of its sugar content.

The drug list of the woman who had a history of deep vein throm-bosis, smoked and was overweight revealed that she was being prescribed the contraceptive pill; she was also in her 40s. Other methods of contraception were discussed with her and her staff member away from the main group.

Benefits of exercise

In the first programme a short, lively video involving well-known celebrities, thought bound to catch attention, was shown. People ignored it. They talked over it, and some got up and walked around. For future programmes, people gained more from talking about the exercise they took and ways of increasing their activity.

Stress

Stress is another topic that often took two sessions, clearly linking to the relaxation and physical activity components. Discussions include people stating what they think stress is and what particular incidents or situations make them feel stressed. A particularly successful activity is to help people to identify how stress affects their own body. This can be done by drawing a body on a large piece of paper on the floor (volunteers being used as template and scribe). People are then asked to make their mark on the body outline showing where in the body they feel stress. Non-verbal people found this a particularly useful activity. Some people indicated stressed parts of their body by touch rather than marking inside the body outline. In two programmes, the following week's health topic was self-esteem, which built upon the issues of stress and how people may be able to reduce stress by improving their self-esteem.

Cancer prevention

This topic was chosen on two programmes and approached in two different ways. The first programme addressed how to protect oneself in the sun. The course took place in the middle of summer; hats were worn and sun creams tried, identifying the best sunscreen factor for each person.

Another programme explored self-examination. Plastic breast and testicular models were borrowed from the HEA, and participants were shown on these models how to undertake self-examination. Men and women were divided into two groups for this session. This approach proved successful for women participants but was embarrassing for the one man who attended. He eventually opted out, possibly because he was the only man.

Alcohol

The LAY approach to alcohol education gives information about alcohol measures and safe levels to drink. Unlike in the group reported by Lindsay *et al.* (1992), few programme participants drank alcohol regularly, so this was not a topic chosen by all groups. Earlier programmes included alcohol as a topic, discussing which drinks were alcoholic, the effects of alcohol and demonstrating the volumes of different alcoholic drinks equal to one measure. Later programmes focused on the range of non-alcoholic drinks available. In addition to 'soft' drinks, non-alcoholic beer and wine were tasted and their cost and availability identified. People were extremely interested in the availability of these drinks as most people did not know of their existence. One newly engaged woman took wine, remaining from a session, home to celebrate with her fiancé.

Clients attending these programmes obviously had different drinking habits from those of the group described by Lindsay *et al.* They tended to live in accommodation with high support. For both groups, however, the knowledge surrounding the choices available was poor. Both Lindsay *et al.* (1992) and McMurran and Lismore (1993) provide further guidance for health promoters wishing to explore this topic in greater depth.

Sleep

Sleep, as identified by Storey *et al.* in Chapter 9, is an important health topic to which little attention has been paid, particularly for adults with learning difficulties. One group chose this topic, information being given about sleep, individual sleep requirements and the influence of medication. It was followed by a discussion about who had sleep problems and ways to approach such a problem using relaxation and physical activity skills learnt on the programme. At the end of the session, one person reported the long-term use of sleeping tablets and the inability to come off them. Support was provided confidentially.

Signs and symptoms of being unwell

This topic 'How do you know whether you are unwell?' was slotted into one of the later programmes run with the community nurse because people requested it. Through brainstorming, discussion and pointing, symptoms were identified and an arrow placed on a body drawn on the flipchart. Serious symptoms such as a high temperature, severe pain, lumps, and symptoms existing over a long time, for example diarrhoea or constipation, were highlighted. The appropriate action was discussed, including telling a general practitioner, carer or chemist, or taking rest and noticing your body and any further changes.

Dental care and back care

Both of these topics were introduced to the two programmes run with the community nurse. The Dental Health Promotion Officer and the physiotherapist led these health topics, which proved extremely popular. A video was used in the first dental health session, but was found to be too complicated a method for teaching toothcare. Therefore, it was abandoned in the second session. Oral hygiene and checking for mouth ulcers were discussed. The dentist considered each person's individual needs and checked that he or she regularly visited a dentist.

The physiotherapist discussed reasons for looking after the back, demonstrating safe lifting techniques, exercises to strength the back and safe sitting positions. Each person was helped to find a sitting position that would be more beneficial, this being reinforced throughout the programme. Programme participants particularly enjoyed having new people to lead the health topic discussion.

Evaluation game

Formal evaluation was not undertaken for all seven programmes. It was, however, included in the two programmes run with the community nurse, in the form of a quiz on the last week, which established what people remembered. In each case, a quiz was designed by programme participants based on questions from the programme content. One evaluation coincided with 'La Tour', a large cycling event that ended in Portsmouth. The quiz was laid out in a board game model with people moving around the 'La Tour' circuit with forfeits such as missing a go for unhealthy behaviour around the course. This type of evaluation was enjoyed, and the majority of questions were answered correctly.

Recommendations for the future

While programmes delivered in this way appear to be a useful means of health promotion for people with learning difficulties, issues were raised that need addressing.

For any form of health promotion to be effective for people using learning disability services, staff support is necessary and staff education and communication links need improvement. Clients are poorly informed about their health status, which compromises their ability to make healthy lifestyle choices. The general public may arguably be in a similar position with regard to information. Staff frequently lacked relevant knowledge about clients' health status, this being worrying where staff worked for the NHS. Participating staff gained knowledge and skills. Their level of ability would not have been adequate to enable healthy lifestyles for clients or themselves prior to programme attendance.

Information sources about healthy lifestyles and hence teaching aids are not aimed at adults with learning difficulties. Few are available, although the HEA has compiled a resource catalogue (HEA, 1995). In addition, they should be considered when any national media campaign is launched or legislation passed regarding health information. Work should also be undertaken to design appropriate resources.

People with learning difficulties should be encouraged to access leisure and sports facilities as a means of increasing both activity levels and community participation. If this is considered too expensive, free activities such as local running clubs and rambling associations are available.

Reflection caused an awareness that the initial attendance on programmes possibly amounted to imposition rather than informed consent to participate on the part of the majority of service consumers. This is because although material inviting people to participate gave a comprehensive explanation of the content and aims of the programmes, it was all written, and few service consumers could read. The use of written material in this way was socially iatrogenic, making people with learning difficulties dependent on their staff for access to information.

It seems likely that the service consumers' motivation for attendance arose from wanting some social activity, or from service providers considering the programmes to be a form of free day care, rather than from anyone's wish to discover healthy lifestyle options. Service consumers ultimately showed a strong commitment to the programmes. Unfortunately, however, their reasons were not objectively evaluated. Obvious enjoyment derived by all service consumers from programme attendance, and the occurrence of positive lifestyle change for some people, strengthens confidence in advocating this approach to health promotion.

A model such as that of the LAY programme fits well with the principles and philosophy of *Our Healthier Nation* (DoH, 1998) and *Signposts for Success* (Lindsey, 1998). A well planned initiative such as this is unlikely to be ignored by the local commissioners and planners of health improvement programmes. Partnerships between education, health, social services, voluntary agencies, residential services, day services, work placement schemes, leisure services, advocacy and self-advocacy schemes could locally develop courses and staff training around such a healthy lifestyle course. A course designed with people with learning difficulties executed in the most appropriate venues over a longer period of time, for example 1 or more years, is more likely to help people to learn skills. In addition, a commitment to individuals having support to practise and consolidate their skills and make choices in lifestyle behaviours in their home and daytime activities is essential. Staff training and resources remain necessary in order to execute top-quality courses. Networking nationally remains a top priority in order to share good practice and prevent the reinvention of the wheel.

Checklist for action

- Programmes should be designed that are specifically aimed at enabling health promotion for people with learning difficulties but that allow integrated participation with other members of the community.
- Programmes should be run in 'healthy living' centres and should promote social integration.
- All programmes should be appropriately validated and involve the HEA to ensure that contemporary, evidence-based methods and information are used.
- The evaluation of programmes should be linked to monitoring *Our Healthier Nation* targets.
- Programmes could be considered as an ideal structure for promoting the Active for Life campaign.
- Resources and teaching methods should be shared nationally through identified communication channels.
- Colleges of further and/or higher education could run health promotion courses for people with learning difficulties.

References

Department of Health. *Our Healthier Nation: A Contract for Health.* (London: Stationery Office, 1998).

Department of Mental Health Sciences. Conference *Enabling People with Learning Disabilities To Use the Health Service*. (St George's Hospital Medical School, London, October 1995).

Greenhalgh, L. *Well Aware: Improving Access to Health Information for People with Learning Difficulties*. (Anglia: NHS Executive, 1994).

Health Education Authority. *Look After Yourself: Tutor's Manual*. (London: HEA, 1994a).

Health Education Authority. *Introducing the National Food Guide: The Balance of Good Health*. (London: HEA, 1994b).

Health Education Authority. *Health-related Resources for People with Learning Difficulties*. (London: HEA, 1995).

Lindsay, W., Allan, R., Quinn, K. and Smith, A. 'The art of positive drinking.' *Nursing Times*, **88**(25)(1992): 46–8.

Lindsey, M. *Signposts for Success in Commissioning and Providing Health Services for People with Learning Disabilities*. (Wetherby: DoH, 1998).

McMurran, M. and Lismore, K. 'Using video-tapes in alcohol interventions for people with learning disabilities: an exploratory study.' *Mental Handicap*, **21**(1993): 29–31.

4

LEARNING DISABILITY COMMUNITY NURSING:

ADDRESSING EMOTIONAL AND SEXUAL HEALTH NEEDS

Diana Sant Angelo

In recent years, the context within which registered nurses for people with learning disability work has changed by virtue of government policy such as the National Health Service and Community Care Act 1990, the introduction of NHS Trusts, and the closure of long-stay hospitals. Social services departments now have the lead role in providing social care services. As NHS Trusts have developed their focus on 'health business', there has been an examination of the activities being performed by community nurses for people with learning difficulties. The nurse has a strong professional grounding in a training particular to people with learning difficulties, and this can be built on to define a health specific role.

This chapter focuses on nursing practice that addresses the emotional and sexual health needs of people with learning difficulties. This area of practice has not been acknowledged in Department of Health (DoH) publications such as the guide that resulted from the learning disability nursing project (1995a). This low profile may be because nurses themselves have not seen the importance of the emotional and sexual health needs of people with learning difficulties in relation to overall health, or of how they as nurses can work with these needs.

This author suggests that the emotional and sexual health of people with learning difficulties has been under-recognised and is a much-needed area of community nursing practice. Underpinning the nursing practice described in this chapter is a belief that there are aspects of the life experiences of people with learning difficulties that adversely impinge on health and wellbeing.

This is acknowledged in the Green Paper *Our Healthier Nation* (DoH, 1998) and described in greater detail in *Signposts for Success* (Lindsey, 1998).

Life experiences of people with learning difficulties that may compromise health and wellbeing

There are features of the lives of people with learning difficulties that, although not unique to them as a group, may present significant difficulties for their achieving emotional and sexual wellbeing (Table 4.1).

Table 4.1   Life experiences of people with learning difficulties that may compromise health

A high incidence of sexually abusive experiences
Multiple experiences of bereavement and loss
Difficulties in talking about their emotions
Limited sex education
Limited expectations and low self-esteem
A lack of assertiveness about sex and relationships
A lack of privacy

Sexual abuse

Research indicates that people with learning difficulties have a higher risk of experiencing sexual abuse. The Turk and Brown incidence survey (1993) found that almost half (42 per cent) of the perpetrators of sexual abuse were other people with learning difficulties, and that most (95 per cent) of the perpetrators were known to the victims, these including family members and care staff. *The Health of the Nation* strategy for people with learning difficulties acknowledged that 'there is an increased incidence of abusive sexual experiences' (1995b, p. 26), and, adding to this *Signposts for Success* (Lindsey, 1998, p. 10), states that 'People with learning disabilities are at greater risk of all forms of abuse because of their vulnerability.' That said, neither document identifies the effects of abuse in terms of the mental and emotional damage done to survivors (Table 4.2).

Table 4.2   Possible long-term effects of sexual abuse

Low self-esteem
Low self-confidence
Poor mental health, for example depression and anxiety
Socially unacceptable behaviour such as running away
Physical and verbal aggression
Self-harm
Poor social skills
Difficulties with trust and conversely an overfamiliarity in relationships, which increases vulnerability

For some individuals, the effects of sexual abuse profoundly compromise their ability to live a healthy life in terms of their sexuality, mental wellbeing and social functioning.

A key reason for the increased vulnerability of people with learning difficulties is their dependent role within relationships. They are in need of help from others and often obliged to cooperate with other people's requests regardless of their own wishes. A person with a disability who lacks assertiveness and sexual sophistication will find it hard to repel the intention of a more powerful person who demands sex. Victims of abuse may believe that they are obliged to have sex because someone demands it; they may be unaware that they should have a choice.

There is a prevalent attitude within society that people with disabilities are of lesser value, and this view increases the risk that abusive people will choose them as victims. As long as people with disabilities are seen as inferior and with fewer rights than non-disabled people, abusing them will be seen as an easy option by the perpetrators of abuse.

The environments within which people live can provide conditions conducive to abuse. Institutional care denies privacy in many ways. People in need of a high level of personal care may have no time alone. The idea that privacy is respected if only one member of staff is present with a person when they are washing or dressing is dangerously naive if that member of staff chooses to exploit this privacy by abusing the client (Turk and Brown, 1992).

People with learning difficulties are seen as unreliable; they are viewed as having poor memories, as misunderstanding or even fabricating events. These negative attitudes magnify a reaction commonly experienced by victims of sexual abuse, which is to have their disclosure of abuse disbelieved.

Bereavement and loss

People with learning difficulties experience loss throughout their lives. Oswin (1991) describes in her research into bereavement how staff choose to diminish or ignore the emotional pain that people with learning difficulties experience when they are bereaved. People are often not helped to understand or express their emotions, and behaviour associated with grief may be interpreted as challenging behaviour and responded to punitively. When someone is bereaved, he or she may have a multiple loss experience; for example, if a carer dies, the person with learning difficulties may be forced to leave his or her home, with a loss of familiar belongings and routines (Hollins and Esterhuyzen, 1997).

One person known to the author was bereaved suddenly and moved to a large care home. She took no possessions from the family home and soon lost contact with her siblings, with whom she had had ambivalent relationships. In the home, she was perceived by staff as rude and uncooperative. However, the reality for her was that over the duration of 1 year, her life had changed dramatically, and she needed to talk about these changes to make sense of them and to adjust to a new life that had more opportunities and freedoms.

When an awareness of bereavement and loss is brought to staff through training from nurses, they start to understand a bereaved person's behaviour and moods as an expression of emotional pain.

Difficulties in talking about emotions

Many people with learning difficulties find it difficult to talk about their emotions, and it is common for an 'acting out' of emotions – people expressing their emotions through their behaviour – to occur. Examples of such behaviour are withdrawal and isolation from others, aggression towards self and others, damage to property, and running away. Such behaviour, currently called challenging behaviour, is commonly understood and addressed behaviourally.

The Tavistock Centre in London has for some years promoted the use of psychoanalytical theory in thinking about people with learning difficulties. Sinason (1990) suggests that people are heavily burdened by their disabilities and frequently also by past trauma such as sexual abuse. However, their emotional experience is often discounted because of their difficulties in talking about emotions. Aggressive behaviours may be seen as symptoms of a person's learning disability rather than an expression of an inner emotional experience. The Tavistock Centre promotes the use of psycho-analysis (Sinason, 1992), a therapeutic approach that is viewed by many as inapplicable to people with learning difficulties because of their cognitive impairment. It is increasingly thought that this client group is able to utilise the therapeutic conditions of psychoanalysis to express emotional understanding in ways that are unique and idiosyncratic but nonetheless valid.

As a starting point for nurses, this requires looking for a deeper understanding of behaviour and emotion, and allowing people with learning difficulties the space and time to communicate their emotional experience.

Sex education

In the past, children who attended special schools did not receive sex education because this was until recently not generally part of the curriculum. The National Curriculum has led to the introduc-tion of sex education within all schools, and this is a positive devel-opment. The previous absence of sex education means that some adults with learning difficulties do not have basic information about sexual anatomy and physiology. Mainstream sexual health informa-tion, for example about human immunodeficiency virus (HIV) and acquired immune deficiency syndrome (AIDS), included in the media assumes a certain level of knowledge and is not fully under-stood by people with learning difficulties.

People may also have missed out on the informal learning about relationships, for example on how sexual behaviour is negotiated, that typically occurs in the playground and after school.

Limited expectations and low self-esteem

The life experiences of a person with a disability may result in poor self-esteem and limited expectations (Brandon, 1990). People may put up with emotional and physical pain because they do not expect that it can be alleviated. People with learning difficulties do not usually ask for help in the way in which non-disabled people do by going to their general practitioner (GP), and this may lead health

56

professionals wrongly to assume that they do not have needs because they have not complained. This problem is acknowledged in *Signposts for Success* (Lindsey, 1998).

Lack of assertiveness about sex and relationships

People with learning difficulties frequently use an 'external locus of evaluation' (Mearns and Thorne, 1991) in relation to their sexuality; this in effect means that in order to be liked they make decisions based on what they think will please other people. They become used to doing what other people say and are less likely to develop assertiveness skills. Passivity in people with learning difficulties may be a preferred option for carers and may be reinforced by them.

Poor assertiveness skills are reflected in people not valuing or knowing their own preferences for their sexuality and relationships, and therefore not actively promoting their own interests. This may result in people with learning difficulties thinking that they are without a sexuality, especially if the significant people in their lives prefer to identify them in that way. Consequently, when an individual becomes aware of sexual feelings and acts upon them, this may be perceived by others as a problem.

People with learning difficulties may experience abusive relationships based on inequalities of power. With reference to women, McCarthy uses her work within long-stay hospitals as a basis for her view that 'Most women with learning disabilities do not have a way of expressing their sexuality that is autonomous from men's sexuality' (McCarthy, 1993, p. 278). It is easy to find evidence of how this results in relationships in which women submit themselves to experiences that they do not like, including agreeing to sex that is painful and humiliating. For many women, the issue of how to form relationships based on equality constitutes a major problem. For men, the issues are often the converse, for example how to form relationships that do not exploit others.

Lack of privacy to pursue relationships

Community care has not given people with learning difficulties a more private life. Many people continue to share rooms in large care homes, and access to the privacy in which to sustain their relationships is denied to them. One woman known to the author described with annoyance that although she has her own room, another resident repeatedly comes into the room when she is with her boyfriend. Other people live at home with carers who do not acknowledge their sexuality and will not agree to their partners visiting them. For some people, this is their biggest problem, and they are being denied a basic freedom.

Community nursing practice

There have been descriptions of the role of the community nurse for people with learning difficulties (Baldwin and Birchenall, 1993; Sines, 1993). *The Health of the Nation* (1995b) provided a new focus for the work of registered learning disability nurses (RNLDs) and was welcomed because it shone a spotlight on some neglected needs of people with learning difficulties. *Signposts for Success* (Lindsey, 1998) provides a comprehensive description of the way in which the current government wants services to be provided, detailing differing responsibilities and roles for agencies. This chapter suggests how RNLDs might work therapeutically with people in the areas of sexual health promotion, surviving sexual violence, and working with feelings. It is this author's suggestion that such work mitigates factors that may compromise health, and as a consequence potentiates health.

Sexual health promotion

There has been a significant growth in this area of nursing practice as recognition has increased that people with learning difficulties have sexual identities. Carers are now more likely to identify whether a person has issues relating to his or her sexuality, and frequently refer on to an outside agency for help. Referral may be caused by feelings of embarrassment or because it is seen as more appropriate that someone who is not involved with the person's daily care addresses such issues. McCarthy (1992, p. 63) confirms the sense in this with the question 'How many of us would want to discuss our sexual lives and problems with the person who is going to be serving our dinner in half-an-hour's time?' Nurses have incorporated sexual health into their work arena, and for some practitioners this is now a central part of their role.

Nurses may work on a one-to-one basis or use groupwork to address the needs of people, and it is necessary to assess what would be most useful for the individual.

An atmosphere of trust and confidentiality within a group is important for participants to feel safe enough to share their concerns. This is fostered by establishing ground rules, by the use of a room that is private with no interruptions, and by the explanation of confidentiality and its exceptions, essentially the need to break confidentiality if someone is at risk from personal harm. Interpersonal skills such as listening and assertiveness can be explored and practised to enable participants to work together within the group as well as to help in their relationships outside the group. Self-esteem can be addressed specifically, and in tandem with this, it is believed that the experience of being in a group where opinions are listened to and respected will be good, and that feelings of self-worth will be enhanced.

The subjects addressed within groups should be determined jointly by the facilitators and the group members on the basis of what emerges within each group. Some issues should be recognised as being too important to exclude, for example the right to say no to sex, understanding sexually transmitted infections and safer sex. Sexual abuse is so widespread that personal experiences of this are almost always disclosed, and adequate time needs to be allowed to enable people to talk about such issues.

Many aspects of sexuality can be addressed in groupwork (Table 4.3).

Table 4.3   Suggested topics for sexuality and personal relationship groups

Personal identity
Self-esteem
Sexual orientation
'Good' and 'bad' relationships
Dealing with conflict in relationships
Being assertive
Body language
Personal space
'Good' and 'bad' touch
Sexual anatomy and physiology
Sexual behaviour
Conception
Sexually transmitted infections
Contraception

These subjects can be addressed in a variety of ways according to the group members' preferred learning styles. Methods include discussion, role-play, the use of visual aids, such as videos and line drawings, and writing. There are many books and resources available to inform the content of group sessions (see the end of the chapter for further reading).

People gain from being in groups in various ways according to their particular life experiences and current relationships. For some, the opportunity to talk about past experiences and to have their feelings taken seriously is of immense value. The environment of the group, with its 'rules', gives people permission to talk because they are made aware that it is acceptable. The facilitator's role is to ensure that the group rules are kept, to attend to the emotional state of group members and to enable the expression of feelings. This can be done by listening, allowing people to feel upset or sad, and finding out what people need. In response to the question 'What can we do to help?', one person in a group said, 'I want you to say that you care about what happened to me.' Another way in which the facilitator can help is by confirming that a wrong was done to the person, for example stating simply, 'It was wrong that this happened to you.'

People can benefit by hearing the opinions of other group members. This is valuable in mixed gender groups for example, when people can hear and respond to the views of the opposite sex. This author has heard men with learning difficulties state stereotyped ideas about gender roles that have been challenged very effectively by women within the group. The women have themselves gained through the opportunity of being assertive in a safe environment, and the man has had his prejudiced attitudes confronted.

Groups of people who work together can provide a self-affirming experience. Opportunities to enable people to give one another feedback can be utilised as they arise or can be built into the sessions. To ask group members to say what they like about each other may sound contrived, but for the man who said in one group, 'I don't like myself, I want to be someone else', it was enhancing to his self-esteem to hear what other people liked about him.

If participants seem to be opting out either physically or mentally, it is necessary to explore how they perceive being in a group. It may be that they have been 'pushed' into the group by a staff member, or the person may simply feel too embarrassed to discuss sexuality in a group setting. If either is the case, individual work may be more suitable. It is the author's experience that if people are aware that their carers are opposed to their involvement in a group, they either decide to keep it a secret or stop coming because the internal conflict is too uncomfortable.

Individual work can focus on many issues relating to sexuality including relationships, 'coming out' as being gay, the use of contraception, HIV, and sexually abusive behaviour. At an early session, it is useful to set a loose agenda with the individual for the subjects that will be addressed in future sessions. The agenda will be influenced by the reasons for the referral, how the person sees his or her needs, and the nurse's perspective of sexual health in the context of the client's life. An assessment of the person's level of understanding can be made as one progresses through the work. It is helpful to evaluate each session and then write a brief plan for the following session, detailing the methods and resources that will be used.

It is useful for both client and nurse to keep a folder of the work done in the sessions, which may be held by the client. The folder may contain line drawings, personal awareness exercises and written work. It is often useful to write down verbatim the words that individuals use to describe themselves, their experiences, thoughts and feelings. Even if the person cannot read very well, writing down what is said makes it tangible and demonstrates that the nurse gives validity and importance to the client's communication, which is of therapeutic value within the relationship. It is useful to refer back to what the person has said in sessions because it assists learning; it can illustrate to the client and the nurse what the client has remembered and how he or she has progressed over several sessions.

Nurses need to be aware of not presenting an exclusively heterosexual view of sexuality. In the author's experience, people with learning difficulties are open to talking about homosexuality and bisexuality, and interested in understanding the meaning of words used to describe sexual orientation. Being gay is for many people a positive part of their identity, and if those with learning difficulties do not know the words to describe their sexuality, they will be less able to talk about it. Workers are wise not to assume heterosexuality just because they do not know otherwise, and it is advisable to talk inclusively about men and women when talking about sexual attraction, relationships and partners. Trust within a relationship will be facilitated if the nurse is able to state specifically that the client's sexual choices are respected and not disapproved of.

Working with victims of sexual abuse

The circumstances in which people experience sexual abuse are varied. The perpetrators of abuse may be family members, sexual partners, acquaintances, friends or strangers. Abuse may be disclosed immediately or years later. Disclosures of abuse may be met with disbelief or indecision about how to respond, or they may be responded to helpfully by carers. Research has indicated that people with learning difficulties want to be believed, to be listened to properly, not to be told off, and to be treated in a kind, caring way by people who are approachable and can be trusted. They have also identified wanting access to people outside their family to talk to, specifically wanting counselling (Simpson, 1994).

With suitable training and supervision, learning disability nurses can work with people to address the trauma of abuse. The use of a counselling approach is helpful, particularly in the formation of therapeutic boundaries to create a safe space for people to express their feelings. In practice, this means defining and adhering to specific times for sessions, and the use of a private room, preferably away from home.

In order to engage the person in therapeutic work that helps the person to move on emotionally, the nurse needs to draw on her own personal resources of warmth, and to communicate concern and acceptance to the individual. Most importantly, the nurse is required to communicate her belief in the seriousness of what the client says because the client will probably have experienced disbelief or dismissiveness in response to accounts of his or her abuse. Believing what the person says may be difficult for the nurse to sustain. Essentially, it is necessary to accept the validity of the person's feelings rather than the factual accuracy of details, which may have become poorly remembered over time or subconsciously changed.

Another useful quality for the nurse is that of patience. One particular woman frequently missed appointments, and often did not want to talk in the sessions. Her reaction seemed to be one of surprise that this was accepted. This behaviour was interpreted as a manifestation of the emotional distress she felt and the ambivalence she had about addressing the pain; in other words, she knew that the pain was staying with her but felt unready to explore it in the sessions.

Mainstream services may be too rigid to meet the needs of people with learning difficulties who may find it difficult to attend appointments at specific times at locations away from home. Lateness and missed appointments may be wrongly interpreted as the client not wanting a service. Learning disability nurses are aware of the needs of people with learning difficulties and can adopt a more flexible approach.

One approach for working with survivors of sexual abuse is informed by the work of RESPOND. RESPOND offers a therapeutic model for working with survivors that is abbreviated as 'Witnessing, Protesting and Nurturing'. The model was adapted by RESPOND from the advocate roles described by John Southgate of the Centre for Attachment Based Psychoanalytic Psychotherapy. Simply put, 'Witnessing' by the therapist is achieved by listening to and believing people's descriptions of their abuse. Sexual crimes usually lack witnesses, and victims may feel that they are alone with their abuse. Workers can demonstrate that they are strong enough to bear to see the reality of what happened. This supports the client as he or she faces the truth about the past. 'Protesting' is carried out by confirming that a great wrong was done to the person, and by helping the person to deal with feelings such as anger about that wrong. 'Nurturing' the person is achieved by creating a safe and pleasant environment, by providing activities to promote self-esteem and personal growth, and most importantly through the personal warmth and empathy of the counsellor (RESPOND, 1994; Corbett, 1996).

One of the tenets of any psychotherapeutic approach is that it is helpful to enable people to identify how they feel. This in itself can be a major task if people have not learnt to identify their emotions and do not have the words to describe them. This problem of limited emotional vocabulary (Conboy-Hill, 1992) is not unique to people with learning difficulties, but they face the added disadvantage that carers may perceive them as being without feelings, so they may consequently be discouraged, either consciously or unconsciously, from expressing their feelings. People may also find it difficult to describe their experiences in a logical way, so it often seems that what people say does not make sense. In such situations, the nurse may need to look beyond what clients are saying and try to understand the symbolic meaning of their verbalisations, drawing from this ideas of how they experience their world. At such times, supervision is useful to explore these themes.

When addressing these issues, a structured approach is needed in order to make the sessions meaningful. This does not mean that the approach is less person centred but rather that the work is less cognitively abstract, which may cause people to flounder. In essence, the sessions are made more 'concrete' by using art, writing and other exercises that clients can use to express their feelings and validate their achievements. One woman gained great satisfaction from drawing depictions of the sexual violence that she had experienced and then cutting the perpetrator from the pictures. In the sessions, she gained symbolic control over the events that had occurred, and changed the outcome in each situation.

People with learning difficulties may find it hard to access mainstream services such as psychosexual counselling or mental health services. This may be because staff are unfamiliar with people with disabilities and feel inadequately equipped to address their needs. Community nurses are ideally placed to extend the services available to people with learning difficulties by working with professionals from other agencies, such as social services, probation and voluntary agencies, for example rape crisis centres. Nurses can be catalysts for the emergence of innovative projects. The benefits for people with learning difficulties are that the skills and resources from different agencies are combined to create services that would be less likely to exist without a multiagency approach. The DoH (1995b) notes examples of the multiagency approach.

Bereavement work

The author has worked for 18 years with clients and has developed work drawing both on learning disability nursing and counselling experience for guidance. People are increasingly being referred to community nursing teams because they have experienced bereavement and it is felt that extra help is needed. Individual work is undertaken using a person-centred approach, that is, working with how people perceive themselves and their experiences and behaviour.

Conboy-Hill (1992, p. 156) presents a guideline in counselling people with learning difficulties which is to 'Find out what the person understands and believes and use this to tell the truth and help them move forward'.

Trying to understand the person's perspective must be a central thread for the practitioner working with people with learning difficulties. A key aim is to help individuals to formulate their own perspective, which may be achieved by providing information, by listening to and affirming the person's concerns, and sometimes by challenging behaviour that is unacceptable. For some people, the biggest value in community nursing input is the time that the client is given that validates him or her as a person. One man asked on different occasions, 'Have you come far?' and 'Could you be doing something else?'; the author interpreted these as being questions about whether he was important enough to warrant time being spent with him.

Another important principle in working with people with learning difficulties is to listen carefully to what is said and to believe it to be meaningful to the speaker. It can seem that what people say is either trivial, repetitive or ludicrous. An example of this is the middle-aged man who repeatedly asked whether it was acceptable to have a beard. By looking at this from the perspective of what is meaningful to him, one perceives the symbolism of having a beard as a representation of manhood, choices, individualism and also how it feels to cope with conflict knowing that not everybody likes beards. The debate about beards was less challenging for him to explore than more emotive areas of conflict in his life, such as the differences between him and his family about how he should live his life.

Using the ideas of the four 'tasks of mourning' (Warman and Fisher, 1990, pp. 1–17), the aims for grief work are for the person to 'accept the reality of the loss... experience the pain of grief... adjust to the new situation... and withdraw emotional energy from the loss and put it into a new relationship or situation'.

People with learning difficulties may become 'stuck' in their process of grieving. One woman with whom the author worked appeared to have put her life on hold. She was resistant to engaging in activities and would frequently refer back to what would have happened when she lived at home with her parents, who had both been dead for 10 years. She described her current carers as accusing her of doing nothing all day; her response was 'they forget what I used to do at home', implying that the staff were inaccurate in saying she did nothing. This woman needed to re-experience the pain of the death of her parents in order to believe emotionally that they were gone, and she needed to adjust to new experiences and relationships. This was done by spending time talking about her parents and other significant losses, by making visits to the gardens of remembrance at the crematorium, and by writing a proposed inscription for the book of remembrance.

Any work involving feelings can be slow, and the identification of progress is needed for both the client and the nurse so that both maintain the motivation to continue the work. Progress can be seen in many small ways, for example if a person continues to attend sessions (unpressurised by his or her carers) or when a person can say how she feels or talk about painful and happy memories.

When working with bereaved people with learning difficulties, it is important to involve carers so that support is available to clients outside the individual sessions and after the therapeutic work has finished.

Nurses need supervision in this type of work. It can be very rewarding to enable someone to talk about his or her most personal feelings and memories, but the nurse needs to talk about her own emotional responses to clients in order to avoid confusing the client's needs with her own. A common pitfall for nurses is to believe that clients cannot cope and to promise to be available whenever the client wants; such offers usually express the nurses' need to feel indispensable rather than what the client really needs, and reinforce a view of the client as incapable of coping. Supervision is widely recognised as a way of safeguarding the interests of clients as well as increasing the skills of the nurse practitioner (Sines, 1993).

Conclusion

The connection between disability and health is complex and requires an acknowledgement that inequalities exist between people in relation to their life experiences, which impact on their potential for health. The simplistic vision presented by *The Health of the Nation* booklet (1995b) was to make direct comparisons between disabled and non-disabled people. The author contends that it was inadequate to conclude that what is needed to meet the health needs of people with learning difficulties is to make an extra effort to include them within mainstream health services. We need a broader view of health needs that pays credence to issues relating to powerlessness, vulnerability and dependence, and includes them within an ideological base for health services for all people.

Our Healthier Nation (1998) addresses the complex causes of ill health, acknowledging that social and economic issues may adversely affect health potential and that these issues may be beyond individual control.

Signposts for Success (1998) identifies a wide range of personnel within the health and social services who have a role in addressing the health needs of people with learning difficulties. It details the complexity of this network of professionals and how good practice may be achieved. This author welcomes this report, and in the context of this chapter, the recommendation that services should be provided 'that promote emotional wellbeing such as counselling services' (1998, p. 64) should be seized upon by nurses.

Some already have the required skills to work with the sexual and emotional health needs of people with learning difficulties. Those who do not have the skills have the advantage of knowing what it is like to be with people with learning difficulties in a wide variety of settings, and they have the potential to acquire skills by undertaking further training, for example in counselling and sexual health work, and by co-working with colleagues from other agencies.

Checklist for action

- It should be acknowledged by commissioners of services that the health of people with learning difficulties is compromised by many hidden issues, for example experiences of abuse, bereavement, low self-esteem and limited life expectations.
- Commissioners and providers of services should acknowledge that people's emotional needs are essential needs that impinge on all aspects of health.
- Service providers should recognise that people are at risk of having their emotional distress labelled as non-compliance or challenging behaviour, and of being treated purely behaviourally or pharmacologically.
- People should have the right to therapeutic interventions that promote their emotional wellbeing.
- Clients should have access to counselling from nurses who have counselling expertise.
- People need sexual health promotion interventions that are specific to their needs delivered by staff with appropriate expertise.
- Training for care providers should be provided by community nurses on issues relating to sexual health, sexual abuse and emotions.

References

Baldwin, S. and Birchenall, M. 'The nurse's role in caring for people with learning disabilities.' *British Journal of Nursing*, 2(1993): 850–5.
Brandon, D. *Ordinary Magic: A Handbook on Counselling People with Learning Difficulties*. (Preston: Tao, 1990).

Conboy-Hill, S. 'Grief and loss and people with learning disabilities', in *Psychotherapy and Mental Handicap.* (London: Sage, 1992, p. 156).

Corbett, A. *Trinity of Pain.* (London: Respond, 1996).

Department of Health. *The Health of the Nation: A Consultative Document for Health in England.* (London: Stationery Office, 1992).

Department of Health. *Learning Disability: Meeting Needs Through Targeting Skills.* (London: Stationery Office, 1995a).

Department of Health. *The Health of the Nation: A Strategy for People with Learning Disabilities.* (London: Stationery Office, 1995b).

Department of Health. *Our Healthier Nation.* (London: Stationery Office, 1998).

Hollins, S. and Esterhuyzen, A. 'Bereavement and grief in adults with learning disabilities.' *British Journal of Psychiatry*, **170**(1997): 497–501.

Lindsey, M. *Signposts for Success in Providing Health Services for People with Learning Disabilities.* (Wetherby: DoH, 1998).

McCarthy, M. 'Sexual awareness.' *Nursing Times*, **88**(51)(1992): 62–4.

McCarthy, M. 'Sexual experiences of women with learning difficulties in long stay hospitals.' *Sexuality and Disability*, **11**(1993): 278.

Mearns, D. and Thorne, B. *Person Centred Counselling in Action* (3rd edn). (London: Sage, 1991).

Oswin, M. *Am I Allowed To Cry?* (London: Souvenir Press, 1991).

RESPOND Workshop. 'Witnessing, protesting, nurturing.' London: March 1994.

Simpson, D. *Sexual Abuse and People with Learning Difficulties: Developing Access to Community Services.* (London: FPA, 1994).

Sinason, V. 'Emotional understanding.' *Openmind*, **45**(1990): 14.

Sinason, V. *Mental Handicap and the Human Condition.* (London: Free Association Books, 1992).

Sines, D. 'Nursing people with learning disabilities: new directions'. *British Journal of Nursing*, **2**(1993): 510–14.

Turk, V. and Brown, H. 'Defining sexual abuse as it affects adults with learning disabilities.' *Mental Handicap*, **20**(1992): 44–55.

Turk, V. and Brown, H. 'The sexual abuse of adults with learning disabilities.' *Mental Handicap Research*, **6**(1993): 193–214.

Warman, J. and Fisher, M. *Bereavement and Loss.* Unit 4 (Cambridge: National Extension College, 1990).

Further Reading

Craft, A. *Living your life.* (Cambridge: LDA, 1992).

Dixon, H. *Chance to Choose.* (Cambridge: LDA, 1992).

Dixon, H. and Craft, A. *Picture Yourself.* (Cambridge: LDA, 1992).

Islington Working Group on HIV and People with Learning Difficulties. *HIV/AIDS, Learning about Condoms for People with Learning Difficulties*, (London: Islington Health Authority, 1990).

McCarthy, M. and Thompson, D. *Sex and the 3R's.* (Brighton: Pavilion, 1992).

South East London Health Promotion Service (West Lambeth). *My Choice, My Own Choice.* (Brighton: Pavilion, 1992).

5

PARTNERSHIP IN RESIDENTIAL SETTINGS

Colin Goble

Most of the literature related to service user participation in general, or specifically to people with learning difficulties, tends to approach the topic with a focus on broad issues of rights and empowerment. Comparatively little literature and research appears to have linked the issues of participation and the health needs of people with learning difficulties, despite the fact that the link between institutional service provision and ill health, both physical and mental, in people with learning difficulties is well established (Greenhalgh, 1994). It is also in spite of the fact that there is an extant literature from within the medical, nursing and psychology fields highlighting the positive effects of service user participation on health and wellbeing (Brearley, 1990). Furthermore, there is a growing recognition that the shift from hospital- to community-based residential care, and thus from a medicalised to a social model of care, has resulted in a downplaying of health issues for people with learning difficulties that, at worst, borders on neglect (Greenhalgh, 1994; Rodgers, 1994; Turner, 1996).

This neglect is not new, but its context and rationale have changed. It must not be forgotten that mental handicap hospitals, administered by the NHS, run by doctors and staffed by nurses, were often physically and psychologically dangerous and oppressive places for the people who were made to live in them. Community-based residential settings will, however, do little better if they fail to address the health needs of people with learning difficulties in the pursuit of some misconceived understanding of normalisation or social care that neglects their physical and mental health needs, and if the change of environment is not accompanied by a radical change in service culture. Beresford (1993), among others, has highlighted the need for cultural change in human service policy and organisation in general, and Greenhalgh (1994) has carried out invaluable work in reviewing the literature and pioneering research into the accessing of health information by people with learning difficulties; her work thus highlights and illustrates in practice important components of changing service culture.

This chapter will focus on the potential for practitioners and staff within residential services to effect cultural change from oppressive and health-damaging, or iatrogenic, practice towards participatory, health-enhancing practice and culture.

A key component in the historical oppression of people with learning difficulties by the medical profession has been their assumption of the powers of definition, diagnosis and classification, on the basis of such criteria as Intelligence Quotient (IQ), adaptive behaviour and biogenetic profiles or syndromes. Theirs has also been the power to determine what, if any, remedy may be applied, and the criteria by which to evaluate the success of those remedies. Taken together, these powers can be seen to have been legitimised by what may be called a 'psycho-medical monologue', in which people with learning difficulties were, and remain, objectified and voiceless. Even when able to speak out, their accounts are given a diminished status, if not dismissed altogether, as incoherent or virtually worthless, emanating as they do from a 'subnormal' or 'disordered' mind.

Attempts by people with learning difficulties to force a dialogue, either verbally or by non-verbal behaviour, leaves them at grave risk of further diagnosis, these behaviours not infrequently being interpreted as symptoms of the person's disturbed or abnormal condition. 'Challenging behaviour' is the obvious diagnostic example, but another, 'relocation syndrome' (Cochran et al., 1977; Bouras et al., 1993), is perhaps more illustrative. It has been used to diagnose what in unlabelled people might be regarded as the unhappiness and stress caused by moving home.

With regard to the health of people with learning difficulties, the consequences of their subjection to a culture based on such a monologue has frequently been disastrous. So steeped is it in pessimism, that ill health is often perceived within its parameters as being normative, frequently going unchallenged, unquestioned or even unrecognised. Also, the damage to health caused by remedies applied on the basis of that monologue remains a scandal yet to be fully discussed or owned up to, let alone recompensed, by the NHS and other agencies. McGee et al. (1987) discuss abuses committed in the name of behaviour modification in the USA, and Wolfensberger (1987, 1990) has of course made much of what he describes as the 'deathmaking' and 'wounding' of people with learning difficulties by services.

However, leaving aside for the present these wider issues, the author suggests that a key strategy whereby practitioners may facilitate a shift of culture within residential settings is the search for, piecing together of and acting in accordance with a participatory dialogue between practitioners and service users. The argument will be illustrated by reference to two case studies undertaken as part of an evaluation of the work of the residential team of which the author was, until recently, leader. The evaluation focused on the use of the shared action planning (Brechin and Swain, 1987) and gentle teaching techniques (McGee *et al.*, 1987; McGee and Menolascino, 1991) on the physical and mental health needs of the users involved. However, instead of concentrating on the systems and techniques used, which are thoroughly described in the sources cited, the focus here will be on the transformative effects on service users and staff of the establishment of a dialogue-based approach to meeting the needs of both.

The case studies used were compiled from various sources, including medical, psychiatric and nursing notes, both current and historical, monitoring systems relating to the behavioural and physiological wellbeing of each individual, and observational records and reflective notes kept by the author. They are primarily qualitative in nature, illustrating both the transformative potential of a participatory dialogue, and the possibility of establishing such a dialogue with service users who have no verbal communication. Names have been altered to maintain the anonymity of users.

CASE STUDY 1
ALISON

Alison is in her mid-40s. At the age of 2, she was admitted to a mental handicap hospital, and there she lived until the age of 39, when she was moved to a locally based hospital unit (LBHU) housing 25 people.

Alison has a severe learning difficulty, no speech (although she has an array of communicative sounds) and a visual impairment (tunnel vision). She is physically non-disabled and very active. She arrived in the LBHU with diagnoses of coeliac disease and psychosis. As a result, she was on a gluten-free diet and various antipsychotic medications. Alison was severely underweight, which was, the team were informed, caused by hyperactivity and poor appetite, and she frequently suffered from constipation. Her menstrual cycle was very erratic, with long gaps between periods that, when they came, were very heavy.

71

Alison's behaviour on arrival with us was very disturbed. She was constantly on the move, walking very quickly on tiptoe all over the building. As she walked, she kept up a near constant, piercing wail that clearly indicated distress. This would intensify when she was approached, spoken to, or touched by anyone else. She became particularly agitated at mealtimes and became very distressed when required to sit down, wailing, banging on the table and slapping herself around the head. She refused to handle cutlery and had to be fed by a member of staff. The only thing she would voluntarily take was tea, which she would actively seek out, grabbing cups from other people and pouring it down her throat in one gulp, regardless of temperature, before throwing the cup across the room.

Alison's case notes from the hospital were very patchy, particularly relating to her physical health and wellbeing, with often months or even years between entries. Her psychiatric notes were similarly very erratic in both regularity and content. The fullest account of her past came from daily notes kept by care staff and keyworkers. These read largely as brief sketches going back no more than 4 or 5 years. Overall, her past was presented in this documentation as a catalogue of problems and disasters, with little that was positive or not related to agitated or self-abusive behaviour.

The intensity of her disturbed behaviour on arrival was initially attributed to the disturbance caused by her move and a lack of familiarity with her new environment and the people among whom she found herself. However, its persistence led to a further exploration of the underlying factors and, ultimately, to a radical reassessment of Alison's problems, both physical and psychological. For the sake of brevity, the outcomes of these explorations and the reassessment will be summarised.

Centrally, the two diagnoses referred to above were both discovered to be unfounded. Her coeliac disease, although it may have existed at some point, was found on investigation to be non-existent, and Alison was gradually reintroduced to a normal diet, resulting in an almost immediate weight gain. The frequency of her constipation markedly reduced, which in turn reduced her level of distress and agitation. Mealtimes slowly became less traumatic for her (and those around her) and she came to demonstrate a clear enjoyment of certain foods, demonstrating preferences that were noted and used to build up a varied, nutritional and – crucially – enjoyable diet. One day, quite dramatically, Alison picked up a spoon and began feeding herself. Here was a skill re-emerging from the past that had been abandoned as her physical and mental state had deteriorated.

The reduction in the level of agitation described above and the concurrent reduction of the attendant distressed and self-abusive behaviours led to an exploration of Alison's psychiatric diagnosis. The result of this was a slow and carefully monitored reduction of her antipsychotic medication, which turned into a 3-year detoxification process from which the 'real' Alison began to emerge, an Alison who could smile, laugh, play jokes, sit and relax to music, enjoy a foot spa and massage, and an occasional glass of wine with a meal. The psychotic Alison, like the coeliac and anorexic Alison, proved to be non-existent.

Alison's menstrual cycle markedly stabilised over the same period, although she continues to suffer premenstrual tension and some distress during her periods. This can now be clearly identified, differentiated from other sources of distress, and thus responded to specifically. Similarly, Alison's sleep pattern gradually stabilised and her enjoyment of a 'good lie in' is now well established and respected.

As well as considering her nutritional, psychiatric and menstrual difficulties, Alison's sensory disability was also addressed, using a variety of techniques and approaches, including alterations to and the enhancement of her environment using contrast in decoration, and the therapeutic use of touch, taste, smell and sound.

CASE STUDY 2
JOAN

Joan's case shows a number of parallels with that of Alison. Joan is now in her early 50s, and was in her mid-40s when she was moved to the LBHU. Like Alison, she had been admitted to a mental handicap hospital in early childhood and knew no other environment or way of life until her move. Also, as with Alison, Joan's case notes and history were very patchy, irregular and largely negative. She came with a diagnosis of psychosis and a fearsome reputation for aggressive and self-injurious behaviours. These included hitting, kicking and head butting other people, hitting herself around the head, pulling her own hair out, head butting walls, throwing herself into furniture, picking and smearing both faeces and menstrual blood, and shrieking. These behaviours sounded, and proved to be, both distressing and extreme in their intensity. More than once, she knocked holes in a plaster wall with her head.

As with Alison, the intensity of these behaviours on arrival was attributed in part to the disturbance caused by her move to a strange new environment. Their persistence alerted the team to deeper seated problems, and there was initially some fear that the diagnosis and highly pessimistic prognosis that accompanied her might be accurate. This stated, for example, that she would never be able to go out, even to attend a day service, let alone to use community facilities.

Joan was also diagnosed as having temporal lobe epilepsy, and, although physically non-disabled, she had curiously deformed fingers. She was also on an array of anticonvulsant and antipsychotic medications. An exploration began into the factors underlying her extreme, disturbed behaviour, the outcome of which will now be summarised.

As with Alison, the diagnosis of psychosis proved to be unfounded in Joan's case. In fact, it was learned that most of her more extreme behaviours were closely related to her physical sense of wellbeing, and a picture of her problems and needs was gradually built up from carefully recorded observations, monitoring and communication among the staff team.

Constipation proved to be a significant factor governing Joan's mood and behaviour. Careful monitoring revealed this to be frequent, and tests and examinations were set up to look for possible causes and solutions. No internal problems were detected, so the emphasis of the response shifted to diet and the use of occasional suppositories and enemas to assist and relieve her of her distress. All these proved highly effective in reducing not only the frequency and severity of her constipation, but also the frequency and intensity of her self-abusive and aggressive behaviour.

In addition, Joan's menstrual cycle proved to be important in relation to her mood and behaviour. Her periods were erratic, although in her case the onset of the menopause proved to be a contributory factor. As with Alison, the identification of the effects of this on her mood and behaviour became apparent only once it had become distinguishable from other causes of distress.

Central to our work with Joan was the reassessment of her self-injurious and aggressive behaviours as being communicative rather than psychotic in nature. Joan, it became apparent, is a highly assertive and discriminating person whose assertiveness had degenerated into aggression, probably as a way of making herself 'heard' in the institutional environment. A process of dialogue was opened up with Joan via the offering of options at every opportunity. Joan's choices and preferences quickly began to emerge. These were recorded and monitored, and the team's response was adjusted accordingly. As an illustration of the subtlety of preferences learned via this process, we discovered that Joan prefers white to brown bread, lightly toasted on one side, and spread with butter rather than margarine. She also likes strong rather than weak tea, and does not like the colour red in her decor, even though she does not mind it in her clothes.

The Joan that emerged was, as was the case with Alison, a very different person from the Joan who had originally presented to us, and the result of this change with regard to her behaviour was equally dramatic. The smearing and picking, for example, completely disappeared, and the self-injurious behaviour substantially decreased.

Joan now enjoys going out, visiting cafés, travelling in cars and walking and rambling in the country, also attending a day service in a local community centre – all things that would have seemed inconceivable when she first arrived. Perhaps most significant of all, however, is that she now actively seeks out contact with other people rather than avoiding it.

There is one final note regarding the results of investigations into Joan's health needs, illustrating perhaps most poignantly the extent to which these had been sublimated beneath her psychiatric diagnosis and consequently ignored. Her fingers, it was found, were deformed as a result of not having been reset after multiple breaks, the cause of which might have been the restraints used in the past to control her aggression.

Discussion

What can these cases be said to illustrate? In reflecting upon this, this author will highlight three main areas of significance, two of which are clearly evident in the case studies as presented, and a third that, although perhaps implied, is not explicitly described. The work of McGee and Menolascino (1991) is of particular pertinence here and will be referred to in this discussion.

First, the descriptions of both Alison and Joan as they appeared on arrival from the mental handicap hospital in which they had lived from early childhood to middle age can be said to illustrate the consequences of a life lived in subjection to the 'psychomedical monologue' referred to above. In both cases, the people that presented at that time were psychiatrised caricatures of their real selves. They had, as it were, become their diagnoses, both physiologically and psychologically, and were both suffering physical and mental ill health as a consequence of their treatment in response to those diagnoses; in short, they were suffering from iatrogenic illness.

Second, the cases illustrate the physiological and psychological benefits that arose for Alison and Joan as a result of having their behaviour reinterpreted as communicative rather than purely a manifestation of psychiatric disturbance. In both cases, their physical and mental health showed a dramatic improvement over a period of approximately 3–4 years.

Third, they illustrate the transformative potential of an approach based on a dialogue between carers and service users. The transformation for Alison and Joan is evident from the descriptions above. However, the transformative potential was equally evident from the perspective of the staff team. As the team entered into an exploration of Alison's and Joan's physiological and psychological problems, they naturally began entering into a dialogue with them. The brevity, inadequacy and pessimism of the historical background of each of them offered only despair for all concerned and led the team into a dialogue, as much as anything, to seek hope that things might improve for everyone involved. As the exploration advanced, so the dialogue opened up and the staff team began to reassess and re-evaluate their own roles in relation to Alison and Joan. McGee and Menolascino highlight this factor in their discussion of the nature of importance of dialogue. As they put it, 'We need to grasp that the person's rejection emanates from a social history that defines us more as instruments of oppression than as companions expressing a helping relationship' (1991, p. 101).

The emerging dialogue became consolidated as both parties began to experience a beneficial change. Alison and Joan gradually came to understand that the staff team were listening to what they were communicating, and the staff team, reinforced by Alison's and Joan's physical and behavioural responses, became increasingly adept at interpreting their behaviour at a communicative level. McGee and Menolascino identify this as a key element in the development of dialogue, stating that:

> We have to read the non verbal communication as much as listen to the verbal. This metacommunication – the combined expression of the person's emotional, cognitive and physical communication speaks an eloquent and complex language. We need to be open to the person's tone, look and movements as well as sounds. (1991, p. 98)

As Alison's and particularly Joan's communicative behaviours shifted away from aggression and towards assertion, the staff team developed a strong sense of solidarity with them and with each other. McGee and Menolascino identify this factor too in their discussion.

> It [the dialogue] helps the person imagine and articulate what a just and equal relationship and life condition might consist of. It expresses sentiments related to safety and security, the goodness of doing things together, and the centrality of valuing and being valued. (1991, p. 94)

One manifestation of this was that the staff team became energised into seeking knowledge and support to help them to help Alison and Joan, for example in the areas of nutrition and visual impairment. They also became strong advocates for Alison and Joan, pushing for action on their behalf from the team leader and higher service managers. This factor is also identified by McGee and Menolascino, who state that 'Dialogue is the energising force of care... It resignifies the relationship by placing ongoing valuing and sharing at the centre of all interactions' (1991, p. 93).

In summary, the establishment of a participatory dialogue facilitated a cultural shift within the service setting, the outcome of which was a significant improvement in relationships between all involved. It also produced a significant improvement in the physiological and mental health and wellbeing of Alison and Joan.

It is important to state in conclusion that, even with the improvement in the health and wellbeing of Alison and Joan described above, they and many others like them still live lives that are qualitatively well short of those which would be acceptable to non-disabled citizens. Emerson and Hatton (1994) have surveyed research on the quality of life in community-based residential settings for people with learning difficulties and make just this point in their findings.

It is also important to remain aware that the 'tentacles' of medical control can, and still do, work their way into community-based residential services, to the detriment of service users. Collins (1993) investigates this persistence of medical control in residential services and highlights it as a significant cause for concern.

There is thus little room for self-congratulation or complacency among service providers, planners or purchasers, and it has certainly not been this author's intention to engage in that here. It should also be stated that the positive outcomes outlined in the cases above were the result of the hard work, commitment and imagination of many others besides this author. They do, however, illustrate the culturally transformative potential of a practice based on participatory dialogue, and this author would offer this as one among the various strategies needed to facilitate the participation of people with learning difficulties as service users, while remaining aware that for the Alisons and Joans in our society, true empowerment lies well beyond what current services are able to provide.

Checklist for action

- Prioritise health care as an essential component of good social care for people with learning difficulties.
- Recognise the benefits to health arising from service user participation.
- Recognise the need for, and develop a commitment to, a shift of culture in service settings, from one based on a psychomedical monologue to one based on participatory dialogue.
- Identify and develop strategies for facilitating the development of a participatory dialogue between service users and staff.

References

Beresford, P. 'A programme for change: current issues in user involvement and empowerment', in Beresford, P. and Harding, T. (eds) *A Challenge to Change: Practical Experiences of Building User-Led Services.* (London: National Institute for Social Work, 1993, pp. 9–29).

Bouras, N., Kon, Y. and Drummond, C. 'Medical and psychiatric needs of adults with a mental handicap.' *Journal of Intellectual Disability Research,* **37**(2)(1993): 177–82.

Brearley, S. *Patient Participation: The Literature.* (London: Scutari Press/RCN, 1990).

Brechin, A. and Swain, J. *Changing Relationships: Shared Action Planning With People with a Mental Handicap.* (London: Harper & Row, 1987).

Cochran, H., Sran, P.K. and Grace, A.V. 'The relocation syndrome in mentally retarded individuals.' *Mental Retardation,* **15**(1977): 10–12.

Collins, J. *The Resettlement Game: Policy and Procrastination in the Closure of Mental Handicap Hospitals.* (London: Values into Action, 1993).

Emerson, E. and Hatton, C. *Moving Out: The Impact of Relocation from Hospital to Community on the Quality of Life of People with Learning Difficulties.* (London: HMSO, 1994).

Greenhalgh, L. *Improving Access to Health Information for People with Learning Difficulties.* (Anglia and Oxford Regional Health Authority, 1994).

McGee, J. and Menolascino, F. *Beyond Gentle Teaching: A Nonaversive Approach to Helping Those in Need.* (London: Plenum Press, 1991).

McGee, J., Menolascino, F., Hobbs, F.J. and Menousek, P.E. *Gentle Teaching: A Non-Aversive Approach to Helping Persons with Mental Retardation.* (New York: Human Sciences Press, 1987).

Rodgers, J. 'Primary health care provision for people with learning difficulties.' *Health and Social Care in the Community,* **2**(1)(1994): 11–17.

Turner, S. 'Healthy bodies, healthy minds.' *Community Care,* 5–10 January (1996): 24–5.

Wolfensberger, W. *The New Genocide of Handicapped and Afflicted People.* (New York: Training Institute for Human Services, Syracuse University, 1987).

Wolfensberger, W. 'A most critical issue: life or death.' *Changes: An International Journal of Psychology and Psychotherapy,* **8**(1)(1990): 63–73.

6

ANTENATAL CARE FOR WOMEN WITH LEARNING DIFFICULTIES

Janet McCray

Moves to community service provision for people with learning difficulties have emphasised a partnership model between professionals, families and carers. This has been endorsed for women with disabilities in maternity services by *Changing Childbirth* (DoH, 1993) and in primary health care for people with learning difficulties in *The Health of the Nation* (DoH, 1995). The Green Paper *Our Healthier Nation* (1998) and the White Paper *The New NHS, Modern, Dependable* (1997) also present a broader and more inclusive view of health and health promotion.

In 1994, Booth and Booth published the findings of a major research study presenting the experiences of mothers and fathers who have learning difficulties. This has begun to raise professional awareness in parenting. While policy documents and research data provide evidence and practical ways forward for professionals, what they are unable to do is to measure the level of opinion, or value placed on people with learning difficulties as parents, by such professional groups. Acceptance and support in the literature does not necessarily create good practice, while a commitment to principles of normalisation may encounter severe strain in the area of sexual behaviour of people with learning difficulties (Mulhern, 1975).

This chapter will focus on some ways forward for community service workers, such as community nurses, social workers, primary health care teams and midwives, in the development of a partnership model for childbirth. This will acknowledge the moral ambiguity that such interventions might present for formal and informal carers, while seeking more positive outcomes for parents, carers and professionals as part of the process. The content is not intended as an ideal model, its purpose being to make suggestions for support in the antenatal period, an area still neglected in the areas of both practice and research.

Setting the scene

There has been very limited research in the area of supporting women with learning difficulties through pregnancy to childbirth, but this is likely to change with the influence of policy documents such as *Changing Childbirth* (DoH, 1993) and with a rise in educational activity to develop positive practice responses.

Research that has taken place in the area of childbirth has focused on the period from birth onwards and has mirrored the ideological, moral and social movements of the period in which it has occurred. Furthermore it reflects the experiences of parents with learning difficulty who have been institutionalised for most or some of their lives.

In 1938, Penrose undertook a study of 570 women in institutions, which looked at hereditary factors, reflecting the eugenic movement's concern with the reproduction of more imperfect offspring, and the myth that people with learning difficulty would reproduce more children than the ordinary population (Pensrose, 1983).

More recently, a study of 34 married couples, all of whom had been in institutions, provided information about their marital relationships (Mattinson, 1970). In the study, several of the couples had children, although the number of these was below the average at that time for a married couple (Craft and Craft, 1978). This study did begin to focus more positively on people with learning difficulty as people first, although its primary aim was not to judge them fit for parenthood.

Mattinson's work has been built upon by Craft and Craft, who in 1974 carried out a study of 25 marriages in Wales (Craft and Craft, 1976). This work was centred upon the levels of support required by the couples in the study, the type of relationship they had and their level of compatibility. Once again, parenting abilities were not the focus, although Craft and Craft record that six families had children, all being cared for in the family.

The work of both Mattinson and Craft and Craft reflects the changing ideological focus of services and to an extent the impact of the civil rights movement and normalisation (Wolfensberger, 1972), central to which was the belief that people with learning difficulty should have the right to ordinary valued lifestyles and relationships within an integrated society.

In the 1980s and 90s, research activity has begun to address the issues of parenting. Prior to this, studies undertaken had focused on four key areas – heredity and family handicap, fertility and family size, parental competence, and parenting training and child maltreatment (Booth and Booth, 1994) – all of which seemed to indicate the negative elements of parenting for people with a learning difficulty.

More positively, an American study (Whitman et al., 1989) linked the parenting skills of people with learning difficulty with the impact of formal structured programmes of support, while in Britain a major research study was published in 1994 (Booth and Booth, 1994). This work presents the experiences of 20 mothers and fathers with learning difficulties, and offers comprehensive findings to inform practice and policy development, which is drawn upon in the content of this chapter.

Because of the need to address or redress the issues in relation to parental competence, research interest in pregnancy and childbirth has been limited. However, the area of sexuality and sex education has provided some research that could influence practice. A study of carers and parents of young people with Down's syndrome (Shepperdson, 1995), although focusing on the control of sexuality, has produced some useful findings in relation to parental concerns, which is helpful when considering ways forward for carer support during the antenatal period. Equally, Craft and Craft's work in the field of sex education (1985) has much to offer practitioners in relation to the development of support strategies for pregnant women and their partners, who have learning difficulties. A series of books produced in 1995 by the British Institute of Learning Disabilities (BILD) on parenting and children's needs will add to the available information (McGaw, 1995). Developing their original research, Booth and Booth's (1997) study examines relationships in families within which one or more parents has a learning difficulty. The work draws attention to the importance of support. While the focus of the research is postnatal experience, it presents challenging perspectives on notions of parental competence and the ability to be a good enough parent.

There is a real lack of empirical data on which to base practice in relation to the experience of pregnancy and childbirth. The Expert Maternity Group, made up of midwifery practitioners, recommends more research on the choices that are important to different groups of women in society.

Having a baby – key areas for support and intervention

The first principle of maternity services is that the pregnant woman should be 'in control of what is happening to her, and... make decisions about her care, based on her needs, having discussed matters fully with the professionals involved' (DoH 1993 p. 9). This chapter will consider the needs of mothers with learning difficulties during pregnancy, in order to meet or work towards the first principle highlighted above. Key areas for discussion will be parenting rights, staff support and guidance, building relationships and communication. The shared planning of care and teaching and learning will also be explored.

Parenting rights

Although the focus of this chapter is support for the mother and father with learning difficulty from the time of knowledge of the pregnancy through to birth itself, the content does not relate to the period of transition to parenthood following birth. Nevertheless, the rights of prospective parents remain at issue throughout. In the most recent study, researchers have identified parents with learning difficulty whose only child was taken from them at birth or immediately after (Booth and Booth, 1994). They identify the cause of this action as being pressure from the immediate families or intervention by the state. The explanation for this response was a perceived lack of intelligence on the part of the parents, which would affect their ability to provide adequate parenting. In this sense, people are being judged without any space or support to be successful parents.

Such responses may be based on the myths or prejudices of service workers. It has been suggested that professionals and parents would prefer to ignore feelings of sexuality in people with learning difficulties (Craft and Craft, 1985), while one writer claims that professionals would prefer to hide their heads in the sand rather than acknowledge the possibilities of parenthood (Gath, 1988).

Staff support and guidance

Such views inevitably fly in the face of the values underpinning a partnership model for practice (Marsh and Fisher, 1992), within which user agreement must be the key and services should be based on negotiated agreement rather than the values of professional workers (Braye and Preston-Shoot, 1995).

Thus, in providing service provision for pregnant women with learning difficulties and their partners, the need to give effective support for those individual workers might begin with an explicit exploration of values and beliefs by team members. Braye and Preston-Shoot (1995) warn against ignoring values. They suggest that there are dangers in assuming a consensus about what is seen as valued, or trusting professionals to remain objective.

In antenatal support, there is likely to be an involvement of a range of different professional workers, with widely differing beliefs, myths and values about people with learning difficulties. Midwives may be involved to provide antenatal care of the mother and baby, while the community nurse's role will be one of longer-term support. This could involve providing advice and support on all aspects of health care for the family. The community nurse may not be present at the birth itself but may have a well-developed relationship with the mother-to-be. This will result in the need for some honest debate. For while professionals might appear to use appropriate and valued language and responses, which creates a feeling of commitment towards the prospective parents, this may not be mirrored in practice. Equally, elements of communication and liaison that hinder or enhance teamwork could be raised, which may lead to further strain for individual parents-to-be. This is important in the antenatal period, when exposure to public prejudice (Masden, 1979; Booth and Booth, 1994) may be significant when attending antenatal clinics and parent-craft groups.

The combination of public and professional prejudice could increase the isolation of the prospective parents, which may have an adverse effect on the emotional, and consequently physical, health of the mother-to-be. This may lead to an increased reliance on the informal support offered by friends, relatives and carers (Rosenberg and McTate, 1982).

Practical suggestions for staff support

One approach could be the setting up of a team support group. This group could be charged with the development of positive working relationships and creating a consensus for practice intervention. One of the activities of the group might be the development of a clearly written good practice guide. This would be based on current legislation and practice protocols, and used as the benchmark for reflection by the group. As the group's relationship develops and the parents-to-be approach the birth date, strategies for problem solving could be included. An independent skilled facilitator could be used to guide this process in order to ensure that meetings occur, that professional reflection is an inbuilt part of the group's activity, and that a mechanism for feedback to and from the parents is created, which decreases rather than increases the stress levels of all involved.

The strategies outlined above may help to develop competence-promoting rather than competence-inhibiting behaviour in professionals (Tucker and Johnson, 1989). In other words, if staff demonstrate a real commitment based on positive attitudes, they are likely to create real opportunities for competence in prospective parents. Booth and Booth (1994) suggest that the values and attitudes of workers may be as important as their knowledge and skills. In antenatal provision, this would have an impact on the planning and quality of support offered, and the opportunities for the participation of the parents-to-be in the pregnancy and birth plan.

Building relationships

Up to this point, the emphasis has centred on staff support and guidance, upon which lies the success or failure of the partnership model of pregnancy and childbirth. This will be expanded here, looking at the development of communication and positive relationships.

Because of the nature of the work in this practice situation, the primary focus of positive communication must be that of sticking with the parents' agenda or birth plan. As there is likely to be an input from a range of professionals, there needs, at an early stage in the planning of care, to be an agreed definition of what the role of the professional team is, with an outline of their responsibilities and the form of support they will be offering. This should be a written agreement (Marsh and Fisher, 1992).

If the prospective parents communicate by other methods, the use of PIC sums (a range of printed symbols, produced by the Loddon School, Basingstoke, Hampshire) or sign language might be appropriate in addition to a written record. If the parents have additional support from an advocate or friend, he or she might also wish to be present at the meetings when these plans are drawn up.

An implicit part of the birth planning process would be the ongoing development of a trusting relationship. All too often in parenting by people with learning difficulty, this trust has been difficult to gain. There is still much work to be done in this field in drawing a balance between the welfare of children and the rights of parents (Booth and Booth, 1994), and in the research study these authors identified that, of the 20 families noted, 14 had children placed in short-term or permanent care. The parents in Booth and Booth's study had ambivalent feelings about the support offered by professionals, describing it as a mixed blessing.

Some key elements of bad practice would illustrate the lack of mutual trust in professional–parent relationships, notably using the parents' fear of losing their child to gain acquiescence, for example taking advantage of people's learning difficulties by failing to involve parents in decisions affecting their lives or responding to parents' concerns. While some of these scenarios could be blamed on fragmented and inadequate services, there seem to be competing tensions rather than collaboration at work here.

Some examples of good practice that would indicate trust are the recognition of the emotional needs of parents, practical support in developing skills, and the involvement of workers with a genuine feeling or liking for the families concerned. A further key indicator was workers having an understanding of the families' point of view, which was not seen as interfering (Booth and Booth, 1994).

Brechin and Swain's (1987) shared action planning approach offers a framework for establishing mutual trust and setting ground rules for the worker–family relationship. Part of the process of developing a shared action planning approach would be determining the boundaries of the relationship and being consistent about these. Any pregnant woman is likely to be anxious and require information about a range of forthcoming situations, not least the process of birth itself. To be unable to ask such questions because of a fear of being judged as incompetent or unintelligent, because it would have an adverse effect on the future of the family, is hardly the basis for her being in control of her care.

Consequently, professional input should work toward mutually agreed, identifiable goals, based on competency-promoting support. In pregnancy, this might broadly relate to practical training in preparation for birth and the immediate postnatal period, counselling that acknowledges any feelings surrounding 'disability' that the prospective parents might seek to explore, and relaxation, together with techniques of stress management.

Langan *et al.*, in their 1993 research, describe some of the problems that may exist in providing sexual health screening and examination for women with learning difficulties. They report that unfamiliarity with procedures and techniques may make an intimate examination very distressing. In routine antenatal checks and in preparing for birth itself, such activity may occur frequently, so an emphasis on the development of relaxation skills should be seen as a priority. A further means of decreasing stress lies in helping the prospective parents to develop systems of formal and informal support. Equally, the needs of the partner (if he is involved) in relation to all of the above should be taken into account. More practically, welfare issues such as housing and social security benefits may need to be addressed at this stage.

Relevant methods of communication

Professional workers may need to plan intervention in a more structured way in order to support people who use alternative methods of communication. This might take more time because of thoroughly checking out verbal and non-verbal cues. When people are familiarising themselves with and learning a new language, for example in relation to pregnancy and childbirth, the use of visual symbols might be helpful. Although these are not currently manufactured for childbirth, workers could design, pilot and make their own. The BILD's series of books, (McGaw, 1995) may be a useful source of information.

Alternatively, if people use Makaton or sign language, workers will need to familiarise themselves with such systems. If an individual has an advocate, communication might be enhanced by their being present during meetings or other activities. Where an informal carer or relative is involved in support meetings, it is essential to ensure that all the communication is not directed at them. Similarly, as Booth and Booth (1994) warn, if the partner does not have a learning difficulty, do not allow him to make all the choices in relation to the birth plan.

Shared planning of care

Setting in place frameworks for value-based practice helps to build the foundations for a shared planning of care. One practice-based approach to care might be the adaptation of a shared action planning approach (Brechin and Swain, 1987). This approach focuses on the equality of the worker–service user relationship, aiming for control by the person with a learning difficulty. Shared action planning could involve a whole range of professionals and/or informal carers as well as the person with a learning difficulty and/or their advocate. Alternatively, it could encompass just one or two individuals and the prospective parent(s)-to-be. What this approach provides is a structured plan with set goals after an exploration of the areas and the ways forward. Shared action planning is usually focused on three key areas – living arrangements, education, and work and leisure – although it would provide a clear way forward for planning pregnancy and childbirth, based on equality and participation.

An alternative, more informal approach is a circle of support. This 'circle' consists of a group of informal carers who provide a range of support to individuals living in the community (Ward, 1995). Meetings are held regularly, and both carers and the individual with learning difficulties are present. Formal notes of discussion and actions are taken. Although this approach has not been designed to support people through pregnancy, it could provide close-knit support, with feedback to professionals coordinated by a link person or coordinator. In some circumstances, intervention from a coordinator or link worker could be provided.

Coates (1993) reasons that, for some prospective parents, professionals and statutory services cannot meet all their needs. He recommends the use of a coordinator with experience of learning difficulty, who could link with other professionals and provide practical support and advice. Coates suggests that the role of coordinator could also be educative in supporting professionals who have some knowledge of people with learning difficulties. In this role, they might take on the independent facilitator brief outlined earlier in this chapter.

Alternatively, the recruitment of a citizen advocate may be beneficial. A citizen advocate is an independent person who provides a means of communication between the person with learning difficulties and others, particularly in the decision making process or where key choices have to be made. The role can be formal and consequently paid, or informal and voluntary. During the antenatal and birthing periods, the advocate would provide the bridge between the professionals and the women concerned. This sounds like an ideal model for providing a highly woman-centred approach. The advocate role could, however, potentially be stressful and problematic, and advocates may need to plan and receive additional support and help, both practically, if their knowledge of pregnancy and childbirth is limited, and emotionally as supporting someone through pregnancy and childbirth could trigger a range of personal issues.

Finally, the positive role of a benefactor is identified (Booth and Booth, 1994). In situations where families have managed to be successful and keep the parents and child together, a crucial factor is the presence of another adult to give support and practical help. Edgerton's definition of a benefactor is 'someone without learning difficulties [who] helps with the practical difficulties of coping with everyday problems' (1967, p. 599). When applied to pregnancy and childbirth, support in terms of attending clinics, maintaining good health and preparing for birth would all enhance the mother and child's care and work toward the partnership model.

Looking forward

A partnership model may mean that workers will need to rethink their methods as well as their values in relation to intervention. This might need to include a review of their role in relation to assessment and problem solving in practice (Marsh and Fisher, 1992), first in establishing a shared model of care. If social workers are to be central to part of this support, some of the potential difficulties of being an 'enabler' and in a statutory policing role might need to be explored (Booth and Booth, 1994) as these could have a real impact on the quality of the partnership model adopted.

Second, decisions about the focus of support and aspects of training for parenting and birth should occur together with the mother-to-be, her partner, and advocates or family. These should not be founded on a 'blanket approach', every possible problem being explored in order to justify the professional role. A more positive approach might be the use of a systematic, structured plan in preparation for parenting. The learning of new skills is more likely to be effective when they are taught in clearly defined, small steps (Booth and Booth, 1994). There is a greater chance of success when the partnership model supports both parents and workers at the same time.

Underpinning this model is the broader and more complex role of the statutory organisations and the managerial frameworks set in place to support staff. People currently have to change to meet prevailing customs, attitudes and standards in society, rather than focusing on the need for society to change to meet their needs (Ryan and Thomas, 1987). Furthermore, changing practice is not only about educating those in practice, but also about changing systems in which those workers operate (Booth and Booth, 1994). Taking into account the dissonance that practice in this area can create, the following sections offer some practical support.

Teaching and learning support strategies

The pregnant woman will have her own views on the amount of information she requires about her changing bodily state and the stages of pregnancy that she is likely to experience. Plans for labour itself will also be made and amended throughout the pregnancy. The following suggested support strategies cannot take into account the individual needs and circumstances of each woman and her partner, so they are presented as a set of general ideas.

Much of the literature concerning parents with learning difficulties draws attention to the particular problem that this presents in teaching skills, notably a failure to generalise learning, and cognitive limitations (Whitman et al., 1989). These problems could also affect the mothers' period of pregnancy and childbirth itself. Nevertheless, research has shown that training in practical skills in the areas of sexuality and parenting can show good results (Tymchuk et al., 1987; Booth and Booth, 1994). However, while a structured educational programme may be necessary, it should not be provided in isolation. Support by means of counselling and a more holistic approach is likely to be most appropriate.

The use of visual resources can aid in explaining the bodily changes that occur in pregnancy. Videos and other teaching aids might help to get the message across, but these might require further explanation and a checking out of the knowledge gained. One practitioner found that the couples with whom she worked had gained a great deal of knowledge from television (Andron, 1983). This had led to an extensive knowledge about babies born at 6 months or 11 months, ectopic pregnancy and twins with two different fathers, but not about the more usual occurrences.

Bearing in mind Andron's research findings, it may be necessary to clarify truth and fiction. Go through bodily changes step by step; this may well be worth doing in separate sessions. An outline of a woman's body can be used to mark changes during pregnancy, and a mirror for the woman to look at her own body might prove useful.

Part of this process may involve offering support in relation to physical health, diet and exercise. In doing so, provide space and sensitive support for the woman to describe changes to her shape during pregnancy. Many people with learning difficulties feel embarrassed about their bodies (Craft and Craft, 1985). As children, they may have been over-corrected by their parents when touching body parts, and many may still feel guilty about identifying and touching their bodies. Further information on bodily changes might be gained by listening to the experiences of other women. This could happen during attendance at antenatal classes or on a one-to-one basis with the advocate and/or link worker.

Preparing for birth

In preparing for birth, service workers and/or informal carers should ensure that the mother-to-be is involved in the planning of a structured programme for support. Differentiating truth from fiction, this should involve going through stages of labour and birth step by step. A discussion of the probable interventions should take place. A video may be useful in helping to prepare the woman for childbirth. However, the desensitising nature of these should be borne in mind. Women may not directly relate the experience to themselves, and it may be necessary to reinforce the experience for the woman concerned.

Visits to the maternity unit to meet other new mothers may be helpful after formal teaching input has taken place. Talking with women who have just given birth and allowing time for questions may be useful and supportive. This should not be provided as an alternative. When teaching skills, the maintenance and generalisation of new learning are assisted by teaching in real-life settings rather than in just the classroom or the clinic (Booth and Booth, 1994).

Those involved must be prepared to listen to the prospective parents describe their feelings as they approach the birth date. Discussing childbirth and some of the screening processes offered may trigger off thoughts relating to their own birth and consequently their own learning difficulties. Equally, the prospective grandparents or carers may also require additional support at a time when concerns over their daughter's or client's health may cause stress.

Provide space and time for the development of the birth plan and ensure that partnership remains its focus when formal input is being provided by others; it is possible that the plans of professionals could override the needs, wants and wishes of the woman and her partner.

Preparation at home

The mother to be and her partner should be supported to prepare a space for the baby. This support may need to acknowledge the socioeconomic factors facing the new family. The health professional should recognise the additional stress that this can create and the effect that this could have on the potential for success of the family. All discussion should occur in collaboration with the prospective parents, planning a way forward that takes into account the housing, employment and benefit needs of the family. The current research literature (Booth and Booth, 1994) suggests that training for parenting is less likely to be effective if the parents have additional stress in relation to housing or other factors.

The benefactor, advocate or carer may need to plan to spend extensive periods of time with the family on discharge from hospital in order to reinforce care for the baby as established in the hospital setting.

The birth itself

Ensure that the same people are present as for formal teaching sessions and support (for example, the midwife advocate or link worker, and the woman's partner). Those present should be familiar with the birth plan and provide support to the mother in decision making during the advanced stages of labour, when changes may need to be made.

Reinforcing verbal information with pictorial visual aids may help to get messages across during a stressful situation. These visual aids should be the same ones as used in the support sessions and should be used at each stage, before fetal monitoring and before gas and air for example.

The feelings of the mother-to-be in relation to close physical contact by those offering support should be acknowledged. It may be that the woman is not comfortable with, for example, back massage if she has not received pleasurable and warm bodily contact as a child (Craft and Craft, 1985).

Costs and resources

To provide the models of support suggested here could be costly. However, such interventions might increase the likelihood of the parents and child remaining together, and where the Children Act 1989 clearly focuses on the welfare of the child, such intervention must be seen within that context. As Booth and Booth (1994, p. 148) remind us, 'the need for belonging on the part of the children may outweigh any deficits observed in the competence of parents'. Furthermore, in separating mothers and fathers from their babies, the babies are not necessarily at any less risk of neglect or abuse if the recent position of children at risk of abuse by professionals in children's homes, or in some cases with the fostering system, is considered (Ward, 1993).

Conclusion

The support of parents with learning difficulties offers a major challenge to the practice of professionals. In this chapter, the issues raised suggest that to achieve a positive model for parenting in the antenatal and birth periods, professionals may have to do more than just provide practical help. Taking on the ideological issues present, while working within a legislative framework, is both complex and problematic. This is compounded once birth has occurred, as the emphasis shifts from the needs of the adults with learning difficulties to the needs of the new baby, and as all involved look to the future.

What should not be forgotten is that intervention from professionals should do more good than harm, and as Ward (1993) states, since people with learning difficulties will become parents, what we have to ensure is that the challenges they face in doing so are not made worse by the services that are supposed to offer them support.

Checklist for action

- Work within models of care that demonstrate the inclusion of people with learning difficulties.
- Set in place staff development for professionals in the area of communication and counselling for people with learning difficulties.

- Build on multiprofessional relationships in order to develop a formal consensus for practice in the area of pregnancy and childbirth. This should be set within the framework of clinical governance.
- Local commissioners of maternity care need to identify a good practice model for supporting women with learning difficulties through pregnancy. This should be used to develop commissioning plans and strategies.

References

Andron, L. 'Sexuality counselling with developmentally disabled couples', in Craft, A. and Craft, M. *Sex Education and Counselling for Mentally Handicapped People*. (Tunbridge Wells: Costello Press, 1983, pp. 254–86).

Booth, T. and Booth, W. *Parenting under Pressure. Mothers and Fathers with Learning Difficulties*. (Buckingham: Open University Press, 1994).

Braye, S. and Preston-Shoot, M. *Empowering Practice in Social Care*. (Buckingham: Open University Press, 1995).

Brechin, A. and Swain, J. *Changing Relationships. Shared Action Planning with People with a Mental Handicap*. (London: Harper & Row, 1987).

Coates, A. *Developing Services for Parents with Learning Disabilities*, in Parents with Learning Disabilities. BILD Seminar, Series No. 3 (Kidderminster: BILD, 1993).

Craft, A. and Craft, M. 'Sexuality and personal relationships', in Craft, M., Bicknell, J. and Hollins, S. (eds). *Mental Handicap*. (London: Ballière Tindall, 1985, pp. 179–97).

Craft, M. and Craft, A. *Sex and the Mentally Handicapped*. (London: Routledge & Kegan Paul, 1978).

Craft, M. and Craft, A. Subnormality in marriage: happiness and the quality of life among married subnormals. *Social Work Today*, **17**(4)(1976): 98–101.

Department of Health. *Changing Childbirth*. (London: HMSO, 1993).

Department of Health. *The Health of the Nation: A Strategy for People with Learning Disabilities*. (London: Stationery Office, 1995).

Department of Health. *The New NHS, Modern, Dependable*. (London: Stationery Office, 1997).

Department of Health. *Our Healthier Nation*. (London: Stationery Office, 1998).

Edgerton, R. *The Cloak of Competence: Sharing in the Lives of the Mentally Retarded*. (Berkeley: University of California Press, 1967).

Gath, A. Annotation. 'Mentally handicapped people as parents.' *Journal of Child Psychology and Psychiatry*, **29**(6)(1988): 739–44.

Langan, J., Russell, O. and Whitfield, M. Community Care and the General Practitioner: Primary Health Care for People with Learning Disabilities. Unpublished report to the Department of Health. (Bristol: Norah Fry Research Centre, 1993).

McGaw, S. *What it's Like To Be a Parent. Children Need Healthy Food. Children Need to be Clean, Healthy and Warm. Children Need to be Safe. Children Need Love*. (Kidderminster: British Institute of Learning Disabilities, 1995).

Marsh, P. and Fisher, M. *Good Intentions Developing Partnership in Social Services*. (York: Joseph Rowntree Foundation, 1992).

Masden, M. 'Parenting classes for the mentally retarded.' *Mental Retardation*, 17 August (1979): 195–6.

Mattinson, J. *Marriage and Mental Handicap* (2nd edn). (London: Institute of Mental Studies/Tavistock Institute of Human Relations, 1970).

Mulhern, T.J. Survey of reported sexual behaviour and policies characterising residential facilities for retarded citizens. *American Journal of Mental Deficiency*, **79**(6)(1975): 670–3.

Penrose, L. *A Clinical and Genetic Study of 1,280 Cases of Mental Defect (The Colchester Survey)*. Medical Research Council Special Report Series No. 229. (London: HMSO, 1983).

Rosenberg, S. and McTate, G. 'Intellectually handicapped mothers, problems and prospects.' *Children Today*, **37**(Jan–Feb)(1982): 24–26.

Ryan, J. and Thomas, F. *The Politics of Mental Handicap*. (London: Free Association, 1987).

Shepperdson, B. (1995) 'The control of sexuality in young people with Down's syndrome.' *Child Care Health and Development*, **21**(5)(1995): 333–49.

Tucker, M. and Johnson, O. 'Competence promoting vs competence inhibiting support for mentally retarded mothers.' *Human Organisation*, **48**(2)(1989): 95–107.

Tymchuck, A., Andron, L. and Undar, O. 'Parents with mental handicaps and adequate child care. A review.' *Mental Handicap*, 15 June (1987): 49–54.

Ward, C. Verbalisation of practice circle of support for adults with learning difficulties. Unpublished description of support offered, 1995.

Ward, L. *Partnership with Parents*. (Kidderminster: Joseph Rowntree Foundation, 1993).

Whitman, B., Graves, B. and Accardo, P. 'Training in parenting skills for adults with mental retardation.' *Social Work*, **34**(5)(1989): 431–4.

Wolfensberger, W. *The Principle of Normalisation in Human Services*. (Toronto: National Institute on Mental Retardation, 1972).

7

EMPOWERMENT FOR PEOPLE WITH A VISUAL AND LEARNING DIFFICULTY

Marilyn Nash

Vision is the dominant sense and the one that provides us with the greatest opportunity for learning. If we come upon roadworks, the noise of the drill and the smell of the hot tarmac give us some awareness of what is taking place, but it is the sight of the traffic cones, workmen and heavy machinery that coordinates these other sensory impressions. Within seconds, we understand the area of the road being worked upon, the direction we must take in order to avoid it, how much of the road is being dug up and the size, extent and nature of the operation.

Some 80 per cent of all conscious learning and 90–95 per cent of all incidental learning is achieved through the sense of vision. The way in which it works is often unconscious, subliminal. We survey the scene, and almost immediately the visual stimuli are 'received' and interpreted, enabling us to take appropriate actions in response. In order to understand just how important this process is in our development, we need to examine its relationship with the other senses a little more closely.

Vision as a coordinating sense

Vision and hearing

Approximately 20 per cent of visual stimuli inform the auditory centres directly. This affects balance and coordination. It also increases the understanding of sounds, particularly background noises, and aids discrimination.

Vision and touch

Information gained through seeing influences tactile discrimination and increases our understanding of objects, pieces of equipment and so on. Vision also has an important safety function – we know before we touch objects whether they are likely to be hot, sharp or otherwise potentially damaging. Furthermore, attempting manual tasks (such as knitting or assembling a piece of equipment) while wearing a blindfold will demonstrate just how much more quickly and efficiently vision enables us to complete a task.

Vision and taste

The appearance of food enhances or subdues appetite – we often want to eat because something looks good rather than because we are hungry. Linking vision with taste extends our understanding of what we are eating and motivates us to try new foods. Visual cues also help to substantiate discrimination between the main categories of taste – sweet, sour, bitter and salt – and the foods with which these are associated.

Vision and smell

The combination of the senses of vision and smell increases our understanding of the context in which a scent occurs, the visual responses enhancing the perceptions of scent. The combination of visual impulses and olfactory ones can increase our awareness of danger, enhance our appetite, and increase recall and stimulate memory.

Vision and Development

Physical development

Vision aids activity, which in turn stimulates physical growth and development. The learning of many skills is denied to the visually impaired person, and fine motor skills, with their close relationship to hand–eye coordination, take longer to acquire. Sighted people make an unconscious use of visual stimuli when perfecting balance and body coordination. The visual element in moving for a purpose, avoiding dangers and selecting different means of transport is more overt.

Communication

The role of vision in communication cannot be overestimated. One of the primary rules of effective communication skills is the engagement of eye contact – not an easy goal for those who are visually impaired. A person's facial expression and body language may give a message very different from that given by the words spoken – and they are less easy to disguise than tone of voice. Consider, for example, the dynamics of a telephone conversation. How much harder it is to gauge the other person's reactions when you cannot see his or her face. How much more difficult it is for both parties to wait their turn to speak, and how much more easily misunderstandings can arise. In addition, when you cannot see the expression in a person's face, a period of silence is just a period of silence, rather than an expression of sympathy or a demonstration of disapproval.

Self-awareness and social skills

Think of life without mirrors – how soon would we forget what we look like? Would that mean losing touch with who we are? – not entirely, but perhaps with some aspect of our selfhood. Vision promotes our sense of body image. We can use the mirror to work out what colours and clothes suit us and to perfect our body movements and facial expressions.

Visual information gathering also gives us the awareness of what our surroundings are like and what 'belongs' to us, as well as enabling us to find our way around our own and other neighbourhoods. Similarly, vision enables us to determine 'contrasts', which aids our understanding and/or clarity of objects within the environment. We learn much about what is acceptable social behaviour from watching others: it is usually by seeing that we learn what is socially acceptable.

New friendships and relationships almost always start with an initial visual response to the other person and the observation of their answering response. Hobbies and other leisure activities, as well as employment opportunities, are often greatly restricted for people whose vision is impaired.

Mental and psychological states

The visual sense appears to play a role in the development of self-esteem and undoubtedly increases opportunities for self-fulfilment. Visual stimuli can increase a person's confidence for the carrying out of physical processes and tasks. They can provide motivation to achieve a goal, and can give additional clues about the best ways in which to respond in many situations.

Rates of anxiety, depression and stress are particularly high in people with visual impairment (Dodds, 1993). This may be due in part to the isolation imposed by being visually impaired in a society geared to sighted people, which can affect psychological wellbeing.

Vision and health

The relationship between vision and health is a complex one. Health problems as diverse as heart disease, strokes, cancer, AIDS and other sexually transmissible diseases, head injury, infections, diabetes, thyroid disease, rheumatoid arthritis and measles can affect vision. In addition, certain medications and dietary deficiencies have similar implications.

A lack of exposure to light reaching the brain can interfere with the normal balance of melatonin levels, which in turn affects the circadian rhythm (wake/sleep cycle). This is because the hormone melatonin, which is produced in the brain, increases when natural light levels fall. This higher level of melatonin is what helps to make us feel tired and prepare for a night's sleep. Sunlight is needed to reduce the levels of melatonin and thus help us to feel properly awake and more alert (Smyth, 1990). If the brain cannot receive sufficient levels of light because the person is visually impaired, the reduction of melatonin is inhibited. Melatonin also has an influence on other hormone-producing glands, which can have an effect on other normal functioning body systems. In addition, high levels of melatonin can affect serotonin, another hormone, produced in the brain, which is known to have implications for psychological wellbeing.

As vision affects all aspects of our growth, understanding and continuing development, a lack of vision or impaired vision can have widespread detrimental effects. Learning processes will necessarily be different in the individual who has been born blind.

The person who loses his or her sight later in life will have to undergo a major process of adaptation, and the loss of vision will have a profound effect on life and lifestyle.

The combination of visual impairment and a learning difficulty

If a person's development, confidence and social adaptation are affected not only by a visual impairment, but also by a learning difficulty, then, by the very nature of being intellectually impaired, that person is denied the ability to internalise and rationalise his or her situation, thereby inhibiting growth and development. The situation may be also exacerbated by:

- restraints placed upon the individual by additional physical impairments;
- a lack of awareness (on the individual's own behalf) of the loss of vision, or a lack of understanding that many of the difficulties experienced are of a consequence of this;
- the person living/developing in large institutional environments;
- being cared for by people who do not have the appropriate skills or knowledge to offer meaningful help that allows growth to take place;
- being cared for in 'systems' that do not understand clients' specific needs;
- being misdiagnosed or assessed as having a more severe learning difficulty without taking account of the effects of a possible visual impairment.

Each individual's experience of visual loss and its effects will be unique to that person, creating multiple problems in many aspects of his or her physical, mental, psychological, social and emotional development.

In 1979, Warburg found that on the Developed World classification of legal blindness (that is, visual acuity below 6/60 in the best eye), legal blindness is more than 200 times more frequent among children with learning difficulties than among other children (Warburg, 1986). Surveys carried out in the late 1980s discovered that 34.5 per cent of people attending special care day units were visually impaired. Of the more able attendees, 8 per cent were blind, but it is likely that a similar proportion were unable to say (Social Services Inspectorate, 1989). A Mencap national survey carried out at around the same time suggested that 39 per cent of children and 27 per cent of adults with learning difficulties also suffered from visual impairment (Hogg and Lambe, 1988), while, according to (Ellis, 1986, p. 30), the 'prevalence of visual impairment among people with a learning disability is about ten times higher than in the 'normal population'. He continues, 'they suffer from a wide range of visual problems, which are particularly common in people with Down's syndrome and cerebral palsy'.

Mobility can be greatly affected as the person becomes afraid of moving from the safety of the chair, bed or familiar landmark. Posture and balance will suffer, and coordination will be slowed. The person who cannot see what he or she is doing will be slow to develop (or even resist the development of) fine and gross motor skills. The ability to complete tasks will sometimes be even slower, indeed, it will be non-existent. Opportunities for learning and development will be restricted, and the person is likely to experience diminished drive and lack of motivation.

The inability to use vision in interpreting the surrounding world may mean that the individual will lack an understanding of much language and may not be able to develop a comprehensive level of communication. Furthermore, the ability to learn acceptable social behaviours and social skills by observing others will be absent. Interaction with others will be particularly difficult. The person with visual impairment and a learning difficulty is likely to have little self-confidence and a lowered self-esteem. He or she may become 'tactile defensive', inhibiting or rejecting person-to-person contact and/or person-to-object contact, which therefore severely limits the formation of relationships and skills development.

As carers, we may see disturbed behaviour as individuals struggle to make sense of a world that is too noisy, too fast moving and too confusing for them to make sense of their place within it. Manifestations of this confusion and alienation may include:

● antisocial behaviours such as rocking, stripping, twiddling of the fingers and so on;
● self-injurious behaviours such as eye poking, biting and head banging (Ellis, 1986);
● displays of aggression towards others;
● relinquishing control over the self and the environment, with a consequent retreat into a world of 'safe havens' or isolation.

A decade ago, a survey for the NHS found 'a shortfall in adequate training and specialist treatment for mentally and visually handicapped people' (Ellis, 1986, p. 30). Anecdotal evidence suggests that little improvement has been made. This chapter aims, therefore, to put forward some practical suggestions for effective working with people whose learning difficulties are further complicated by the problems associated with impaired vision.

Recognising visual problems

There are three causes of visual impairment:

1. physiological damage to the eyes and their structures;
2. cortical impairment, that is, healthy eyes but damage to the visual cortex of the brain, or failure to process visual stimuli, resulting in impaired vision;
3. failures of motivation: that is, some people act as if they are blind because they lack the motivation and/or ability to use their vision.

Before any interactive work is planned with an individual, it is most important that the person's sight is fully tested by an experienced ophthalmic optician and the type and extent of impairment is assessed. Knowing what the problem is will greatly affect how we care for that person.

Physiological damage can include errors of refraction, that is:

- myopia (short sight): an inability to see clearly at a distance;
- hypermetropia (long sight): not being able to see clearly close up;
- astigmatism: blurred vision;
- presbyopia: an age-related problem in which the lens loses its ability to accommodate for near vision;

and/or conditions such as glaucoma, macular degeneration, diabetic retinopathy and optic atrophy, to name but a few. What is important, however, is that each condition will affect the level of vision in different ways: some will affect the ability to use the 'central' vision, some will reduce the ability to use the 'peripheral' vision, and some will create 'patches' of lost visions. In more than 90 per cent of people classified as 'blind' and in everyone classified as 'partially sighted' some residual vision will, however, remain. Knowing what this functional vision is by knowing what is causing the visual impairment will determine how we can best support the individual to use his or her remaining vision to optimum capacity. It is important to be aware that errors of refraction are frequent among individuals with a learning difficulty. Furthermore, large errors of refraction, which severely affect functional vision and which can be a cause of detached retina in myopic vision, are particularly common among people with a learning difficulty.

According to (Warburg, 1986, p. 93), 'the commonest cause of low vision (among people with a learning difficulty) is lack of spectacles and, since the majority of learning disabled people can use glasses, the prescription of spectacles is one of the cheapest ways of treating a handicapping condition among multi-handicapped people'. The importance of eye tests for people with a learning difficulty cannot be overstated.

In cases where the experience of undergoing an eyesight test might prove too traumatic, carers can help to prepare individuals by enabling them to become accustomed to a darkened room and accept the light from a pen torch:

- Identify a room that you will be able to darken, somewhere quiet, undisturbed and familiar to the person concerned.
- In full light, help the individual to become accustomed to the pen torch. Shine it on each other's hands, faces and so on. Make it fun!
- At a distance, begin shining the light into the individual's eyes (one at a time) and gradually move closer, to within 1 or 2 inches of each eye.
- Practise this frequently while simultaneously and gradually 'darkening' the room.
- Use such phrases as 'Look this way' and 'Open your eyes'.

When the individual concerned is able to tolerate the light from a pen torch in a dark room for 1 or 2 minutes at a distance of 1 or 2 inches from each eye, arrange the eye test. This can be either a domiciliary visit so that it can be undertaken in familiar surroundings, or one to an empathetic optician willing to offer a little extra time. With just this amount of cooperation, the optician will be able to carry out an 'objective test' (Gaston and Elkington, 1986). Where the individual is able to understand and cooperate sufficiently, this objective test can provide the baseline from which to continue with 'subjective testing', allowing a refinement of the prescription to take place (Gaston and Elkington, 1986).

If a refractive error has been identified and spectacles prescribed, the individual may need support and guidance from the carers to accept wearing the glasses and interact with the environment. There may be many and diverse reasons why individuals initially reject their glasses – comfort, fit, not being used to seeing themselves with glasses and so on – but the greatest reason is probably the adjustment to the distortions and magnifications/minifications caused by the power (dioptre) of the lens, creating a world with sloping floors, curved walls, door frames and difficulty in judging distances. The larger the refractive error, the bigger the prescription required, which in turn results in greater distortions, so a seemingly alien world, rather than a familiar blurred world, is seen by the individual. It must, however, be remembered that uncorrected large refractive errors will result in the individual remaining with severely impaired vision, causing not only a reduction in what can be seen clearly, but also an inability to distinguish colours and contrasts, which minimises the interpretation of the environment.

As people with learning difficulties are now living longer, they are subject to the same age-related eye degeneration as the rest of the population. It is important to ensure, therefore, that all people with a learning difficulty have a regular eye test (at least once a year unless otherwise advised) so that any problems can be responded to as soon as they arise. Staff working with this client group should remember that the eyes are particularly vulnerable in people with diabetes, those who have had heart disease or a stroke, those with thyroid problems, anyone who has suffered an accident, particularly involving a head injury, people whose nutritional intake is poor (particularly if it is lacking in vitamins A, B2, C, E and beta-carotene) and people on a complicated medication regime.

The Royal National Institute for the Blind (RNIB) has produced a leaflet which makes invaluable reading (RNIB, 1992). The reader is also referred to *Vision for Doing* (Aitken and Buultjens, 1992), which offers a fuller description of cortical impairments.

If glasses have been prescribed, it must be made sure that they fit properly, are in good repair, clean and accessible, and that they are used.

Learning through the senses

Vision is our dominant and main coordinating sense. We learn about ourselves and our environment through the senses. If vision is impaired, information must be interpreted through the remaining senses. Although it is not actually true that people whose sight is deficient have a better sense of hearing, touch, taste or smell, these other senses do have to be developed in order to be used effectively.

However, many people with learning difficulties lack the skills and/or motivation to develop their other senses to a sufficient extent. Thus, the aim of the person working with those with learning difficulties and visual impairment should be to stimulate the use of each sense through intensive interactions, so that individuals can become increasingly aware of themselves and their environment. In this way, they can be empowered to exert a level of control over their own lives, can learn how to communicate preferences and choices, and can discover how to use their senses in a way that will enable them to grow and develop more independently.

A structured programme can be worked out with the aim of stimulating and developing each sense individually. Activities should be taken one at a time and each activity broken down into micro steps. The smallest stages of each activity, situation and piece of equipment should be considered. The individual will be totally dependent on the professional for guidance on how to approach the activity and every item of equipment needed to carry it out.

If, for example, you are going to introduce a person to the activity of painting, you should begin by considering the equipment involved. Ask yourself, 'What does a paintbrush "look" like?' It must be held and manipulated, the difference between the hard handle and the soft bristles must be explored, the weight and feel of it as an object must be tried out. Try blindfolding yourself and then picking up a brush with one hand. Try to imagine never having seen a brush. Could you honestly judge its length? How would you be able to develop a concept of what this object is? It may be almost as long as you are tall or it may end just beyond where your fingers are holding it. Now bring your other hand into the activity: you will be able to increase your understanding enormously.

If the individual with whom you are working is unable to use both hands together, you should, with hand over hand, physically encourage him or her to explore the object in order to gain some understanding. Then encourage the individual to use the other senses. Does the brush have a smell? What happens when it is put in water? What difference does the addition of water make to the feel of the bristles? To the object as a whole? How does it feel and smell now?

This process is intense and will need to be repeated several times with the brush, the paper, the paints and everything else that is involved. You, as the teacher, need to initiate, direct, lead and control what is happening until a recognition of what is taking place begins to develop.

Acute powers of observation on the part of the carer are necessary to gauge the response. If the individual has severe disabilities, the response may be so small that it could be missed. It could be signalled by a mere flicker of an eyelid, a fleeting change of expression, the smallest movement of a finger. But these can all denote a response, and you will need to have observed them in order to assess your next response to facilitate the movement towards a level of independence. What this process achieves is the removal of the fear and mystery from unknown objects and situations, replacing these with real understanding. Self-confidence will increase with each new situation until a permanent change finally takes place between the person's communication pattern and the relationship with the activity or object concerned. Naturally, not everyone will attain the same level of achievement, because of their own physical and learning restraints. However, a greater depth of learning is possible for everyone when the situation is approached in a way that takes account of the combined effects of a visual and learning difficulty. For detailed information on developing a sensory programme, the reader is referred to *A Sensory Curriculum for Very Special People* (Longhorn, 1988).

In order to consider further the breaking down of experiences, situation and equipment into micro aspects, it is perhaps helpful to consider each sense in turn. Think about addressing each sense, and consider how you can motivate the individual to explore it. Through such exploration, how can individuals best be enabled to understand and interpret the areas of learning that their sighted contemporaries may find so easy through the use of vision?

Touch

Touch is not only a basic human need, but also one of the earliest forms of communication known to humankind. Touch allows us to make contact with others, to express our emotions and to reinforce verbal information. This sense also enables us to comfort ourselves and others during times of hurt, pain or sorrow, and to give and receive love and nurture. 'When we are prevented from touching or being touched, we feel painfully alone and anxious' (Lidell, 1992 , p. 14).

Touch can be divided into two categories (Watson, 1975):

- *instrumental*, that is, perfunctory tasks performed 'for' or 'to' another person – bathing, dressing a wound, giving suppositories and so on;
- *expressive*, that is, giving and sharing in a basic human way, an arm round the shoulder, a gentle pat on the hand.

It is probable, however, that many adults with a learning difficulty will have been denied familiarity with normal expressive touch because of the large, impersonal environment in which they have lived. Additionally, much of the touch they have experienced may have been unpleasant (for example, enemas), painful (for example, injections) or simply perfunctory (for example, help with bathing and other activities of living). Such experience, particularly in the person who is also visually impaired, may well have resulted in tactile defensiveness. This must be overcome before any other skills training can proceed. The aims and objectives for this could then include the following:

- to promote the engagement of the individual in tactile communication and to help him or her to understand the cause and effect of objects and equipment;
- to promote a better understanding and acceptance of personal care (for example, washing the hair, cutting the nails and so on);
- to reduce the fear and anxiety surrounding potentially painful procedures (for example, injections and enemas);
- to reduce the startle reflex, which can in turn cause pain;
- to initiate contact and develop relationships;
- to enable an exploration and understanding of the individual's self-image;
- to accept a wide variety of tactile stimuli that will allow participation in a range of activities, that is, self-care (for example, holding a toothbrush, hairbrush, flannel or soap), daily living (for example, washing up, vacuuming, polishing, or doing the laundry), hobbies and leisure (for example, painting, modelling, gardening and cooking), community presence (for example, shopping, library visits, swimming and outings and education/work/structured day activities;
- to aid mobility by using tactile clues as points of reference for 'orientation', 'trailing' or the location of objects;

- to develop and increase fine and gross motor movements, balance and hand–eye coordination;
- to enable an individual to anticipate 'what comes next';
- to promote the individual's safety both at home and within the community.

Tactile defensiveness can be addressed by using such techniques as 'therapeutic touch', aromatherapy and massage. Benefits and techniques relating to these therapies are discussed in detail by Lidell (1992) and Sanderson *et al.* (1991). However, other contraindications and cautions are listed by Arnould-Taylor (1991).

Mobility and orientation

Visual impairment severely restricts movement and modes of travel. There are also further restrictions on individuals with a learning difficulty, particularly if they are reliant on carers who may not be aware of the correct method of guiding or the implications of wheelchair dependence for people with both visual impairment and a learning difficulty. In many instances, therefore, moving around can be a frightening experience for individuals and one which they may try to avoid.

When considering how best to encourage mobility and orientation in a person with both visual impairment and a learning difficulty, one should begin by thinking of the wider framework and how movement and orientation begin:

- Movement begins when the infant is still in its cot, reaching for mobiles and so on (directed by vision):
- Crawling towards a goal is again motivated by having sight of the goal.
- In toddling, the first tentative steps, the more movement there is of whole body parts, the better that coordination and balance develop.
- Increased feelings of security, with a growing ability to master movement, lead to greater self-confidence and motivation towards true mobility.
- Vision enables running, jumping and skipping to develop through a natural progression, finally leading the individual towards independent mobility.

The author has met several carers who, not understanding either the individual's visual problems or the effects of going out into unfamiliar environments, have misjudged the difficulties involved. Having observed an individual walking about unaided at home, the carer assumes that person is being difficult if he or she stands and screams, refuses to move or drops to the floor when taken out. This is a facile interpretation. Individuals build up visual images of their own – familiar – home, thereby gaining confidence and security to move within it safely. When taken into unfamiliar surroundings, they become much more aware of their lack of vision (even if they are not able to acknowledge for themselves what has happened). This greatly undermines their self-confidence and with it their security. If a person does not have the elaborate language skills to explain what it feels like to go into an unfamiliar, crowded or noisy environment, negotiate steps, kerbs, uneven surfaces and cope with the elements, he or she has no alternative but to communicate in another way.

Guiding a visually impaired person properly is an easy technique to learn and will benefit both the individual and the carer. Enabling individuals to develop safe mobility skills can open up a whole new world for them and reduce their frustration and anxiety. Many will be enabled to go out of the house and into the community in a way that empowers them. Those who 'cling' to the safety of a chair or bed can be offered the freedom of their own homes, greatly increasing the quality of their lives. The basic principles of the 'sighted guide' technique are given below.

Sighted guide technique

1. Make contact with an individual and explain what you are about to do, that is, go for a walk, to the shops or just into another room. (People with visual and learning disabilities are often just moved about and taken places without any explanation.)
2. Stand beside the person you wish to guide and, keeping your arm by your side, ask him or her, or physically support the person, to hold your arm just above your elbow so that his or her fingers are on the inside of your arm, the thumb being on the outside and the elbow bent. This is your 'grip' arm. To give a little extra security, you can cup one hand over the individual's hand, which is above your elbow.

3. The individual should be half a pace behind you and therefore able to detect when and how you are turning, mounting different surfaces and so on by the movement of your body.
4. You are now in the correct position to walk ahead. Ensure that you remain close together: do not let your bodies move too far apart.
5. To change sides, the correct procedure is to ask the individual to slide his or her hands across your back and take up the grip position on your other arm while you remain still. For someone with a learning disability, it may, however, prove easier to ask the person to remain still while you change sides, keeping contact across the top of back.
6. If you need to walk in a single file, indicate this by moving your grip arm over to the middle of your back but still keeping the arm straight, while simultaneously asking the individual to step behind you.
7. If you need to leave the individual you are guiding, always put him or her in contact with something – a wall, a table or, better still, a chair. Never leave someone stranded without the security of something concrete to 'lean' on. Always say if and when you are leaving them and when you will be back.

Negotiating steps/stairs

1. Approach steps or stairs at right angles in the 'grip' position, and say whether it is 'steps up' or 'steps down'. If necessary, change sides to position the individual on the side of the banister or hand rail if there is one. Inform the individual if the hand rail ends before the last step.
2. As the guide, take the first 'step up'; as you do so the individual will feel your arm and body move in an upwards direction. As you take the second step up, say 'Step up' so that the individual takes the first step up.
3. Continue in this way, always being one step ahead of the individual – his or her arm will remain slightly stretched forward and upward. Continue to say 'Step up' until you reach the top.
4. As you approach the last step, take a longer stride forward and then, as the individual alights on the last step, say that it is his or her 'Last step up'.
5. The reverse procedure will be employed for going downstairs.

Negotiating chairs

The person should always be given an opportunity to judge the size and shape of a chair before sitting down.

1. Staying in the grip position, locate the back of the chair from behind, and allow the individual to slide his or her hand down your arm until the chair is located. The person can then negotiate where the arms are and lower him- or herself into the seat.
2. Alternatively, approach the chair from the front and place the individual's hands directly onto the arms of the chair (or the seat if there are no arms). Again allow the person time for getting into the chair.

Crossing roads

1. The guide must always take responsibility for deciding when it is safe to cross, while simultaneously allowing the individual to experience road safety awareness.
2. Choose a crossing point that is away from parked vehicles, the brow of a hill, or any bends in a road, thus ensuring a clear view of the road and the oncoming traffic.
3. If it is a regular route, try to identify a crossing point that will also have a 'tactile clue' (for example, a lamp post or street sign) close by, and then always use this same spot to cross the road. This will help with orientation when taking a planned route.
4. Once you have located your 'crossing point', stand on the kerb and identify the sounds of passing traffic vehicles. Then identify when it is quiet and therefore safe to cross.
5. Say 'Step down' and then 'Walk ahead' as you cross the road. While crossing the road, stop talking to allow the individual the opportunity to use his or her hearing.

Rehabilitation officers for the visually impaired are employed by social service departments. They are highly skilled in techniques of mobility and orientation training, as well as in advising on safety within the home and route planning. The RNIB can also offer comprehensive training on mobility and wheelchair mobility for the visually impaired person with a learning difficulty. They also produce a very useful booklet *How to Guide a Blind Person* (RNIB).

Facilitating communication

From the beginning of time, even before formal communication systems evolved, human beings have communicated with each other. Communication is as much a human need as is touch. When vision is impaired, it is important to make the most of all the senses for promoting, developing and enhancing communication.

At the beginning of any such programme, the individual's level of 'communication' must be assessed with care. The person making the assessment must have good observational skills and also be aware that, in the profoundly impaired individual, the smallest movement or slightest sound may be a deliberate act of communication. The individual's greatest disadvantage may be that we, as carers, do not listen hard enough, or for long enough, to hear what he or she is saying. We often do not recognise that communication is indeed taking place. Such communication as there is must be used as a baseline for teaching a more formal system. Some key principles of effective communication with people who have both a visual impairment and a learning difficulty might be as follows:

- Always approach the individual you want to speak with. Never call from a distance as sound may be distorted, particularly if the environment is a busy one.
- Make full use of the person's visual range and optimum visual body position. For example, if the person has better vision in the right eye, sit on his or her right-hand side).
- If possible, sit or stand with the light falling on your face.
- Use the person's first name (or preferred mode of address) before delivering your message, so that it will be clear whom you are addressing.
- Then say who you are – give your name together with any 'tactile' name or association you may have (bracelet, ring, beard and so on). Combine this with a gentle touch on the shoulder or hand, which can replace a human warmth that cannot be seen through a smile or eye contact.
- Listen carefully to the sound of your own voice: stress, fatigue and other such emotions can communicate themselves if you are not particularly vigilant. Use a pitch that does not imply you think that the person is also deaf.
- Take time: allow the other person to receive, decode and respond to your message.

- Give your message in language that takes account of the fact that many visually impaired people may not understand some of the terminology used by sighted people. Much of what we say only makes sense if we can see.
- If your message consists of instructions to do something, check that the recipient has understood, and determine whether assistance is needed.
- Be descriptive: use all *your* senses to get the message across and indicate (for example, through touch and voice) whether you are taking away a cup of tea, offering medication and so on.
- Think carefully about your own responses. Use interjections that can be heard (rather than nodding, smiling, and so on) to indicate to the speaker that you are still there and still engaged with the conversation.
- Before leaving, say that you are going and when you will be back.

Summary

The combination of visual impairment and learning difficulty often leads to multiple complex problems for the individual, with the potential to affect his or her mental, physical, emotional, social and psychological wellbeing. The Government's recent consultative Green Paper, *Our Healthier Nation*, has identified four priority areas on which to focus; heart disease and stroke, cancer, accidents and mental health. The individual with such complex needs is clearly at particular risk within each of the targeted areas. To ignore their specific needs will have alarming repercussions on the individual's quality of life and subsequent greater dependency on the services.

The needs of this disadvantaged group of people are clearly complex and specific to each individual. This chapter has barely touched the surface of the many and diverse issues involved, but it is to be hoped that it has at least raised enough awareness in the reader to seek further and more in-depth information. The most valuable resource the individual with visual and learning difficulties has is you, the carer and service provider. If you empower yourself with knowledge, you are then in a position to empower the individual concerned towards a more fulfilling and independent life, and above all, to restore a sense of self-worth and the opportunity to live a life with dignity.

Checklist for action

- Provide the staff training, education, awareness and skills development necessary for the appropriate care of this particular client group.
- Identify minimum standards that include screening and accurate record keeping for those people on specific drug regimes, predisposed towards anxiety, stress or depression, at nutritional risk, or most vulnerable or predisposed to other health-related issues.
- Ensure that everyone has access to regular eye tests, with provision for more specialised screening for the individual unable to comply with the full range of testing procedures.
- Provide alternative and more accessible ways to communicate information material around a wide range of 'health promotion' issues, for example healthy eating, accident prevention, safe sexual practices and healthy lifestyles.
- Set minimum standards to provide 'visible' access within the person's own home that will help to reduce the risk of accidents.
- Initiate effective communication systems so that individuals can begin to exert a level of 'choice' and 'control' over their lives.
- Provide structured 'mobility and orientation' programmes, and 'route planning' to reduce the risks of accident and injury.
- Offer access to the appropriate rehabilitation services.

References

Aitken, S. and Buultjens, M. *Vision for Doing: Assessing Functional Vision of Learners who Are Multiply Disabled*. (Glasgow: Bell & Bain, 1992).

Arnould-Taylor, W.E. *The Principles and Practice of Physical Therapy* (3rd edn). (Cheltenham: Stanley Thornes, 1991).

Dodds, A. *Rehabilitating Blind and Visually Impaired People*. (London: Chapman & Hall, 1993).

Ellis, D. *Sensory Impairments in Mentally Handicapped People*. (London: Croom Helm, 1986).

Gaston, H. and Elkington, A.R. *Ophthalmology for Nurses*, (Kent: Croom Helm, 1986).

Hogg, J. and Lambe, L. Mencap profound retardation and multiple handicap project. (Manchester, July, 1988).

Lidell, L. *The Book of Massage*. (London: Ebury Press, 1992).

Longhorn, F. *A Sensory Curriculum for Very Special People*. (London: Souvenir Press, 1992).

Royal National Institute for the Blind. *Looking for Eye Problems in People with Learning Difficulties*. Focus Fact Sheet. (RNIB, 1992).

Royal National Institute for the Blind. *How to Guide a Blind Person*. (RNIB booklet).

Sanderson, H. and Harrison, J. *Aromatherapy and Massage for People with Learning Difficulties*. (Birmingham: Hands on Publishing, 1991).

Smyth, A. *SAD: Seasonal Affective Disorder*. (London: Unwin, 1990).

Social Services Inspectorate. *Inspection of Day Services for People with a Mental Handicap*. (London: HMSO, 1989).

Warburg, M. 'Medical and ophthalmological aspects of visual impairment in mentally handicapped people', in Ellis, D. (ed.) *Sensory Impairments in Mentally Handicapped People*. (London: Croom Helm, 1986, p. 93).

Watson, W. 'The meaning of touch.' *Geriatric Nursing Journal of Communication*, **25**(3)(1975): 104–12.

8

LEARNING DIFFICULTIES AND HEARING IMPAIRMENT

Christine Jenkins and Sue Shearman

Hearing loss and learning difficulty

The fact that people with learning difficulties are more likely to have a hearing loss than the general population is widely acknowledged. The publication, *The Health of the Nation: A Strategy for People with Learning Disabilities* (DoH, 1995), included hearing problems in a list of health problems and disabilities more commonly experienced by people with learning difficulties.

Both hearing loss and learning difficulties on their own have significant effects on the development and functioning of an individual. In particular, both conditions have major implications for communication, affecting the development, understanding and effective use of spoken language, the intelligibility of speech, and the ability to use auditory clues in the environment. However, when both conditions are present in one individual, as Stewart (1978) says, the effect of hearing loss on a learning disability is not simply an additive one but one of 'reciprocal limitations'; that is, a hearing loss makes learning more difficult, which increases the level of disability. The use of auditory clues decreases, which in turn further intensifies the level of disability. This highlights the importance of identification so that action can be taken in order to minimise the added disability of hearing loss. Furthermore, unrecognised hearing loss can lead an individual to display behaviours regarded as challenging, or to develop psychological reactions, such as depression, that require specialist interventions and treatment, as well as limiting opportunities for community participation. There are also resource implications for services, and costs that could be avoided.

The diagnosis of a hearing loss in someone who also has a learning difficulty is not easy. One obvious indicator of hearing loss in young children is delayed speech and language development, and as this is frequently also a feature of learning difficulties, it is all too easy not to recognise that both conditions are present. When hearing fluctuates or deteriorates, people with learning difficulties may be unable to express the fact and describe the symptoms, so the condition may go unnoticed. Many methods of testing hearing require active cooperation, which presents problems for a significant number of people with severe and profound learning difficulties.

All of these factors help to explain why research to establish the incidence of hearing impairment and learning difficulty has historically shown widely differing results. Studies by Lloyd and Reid (1967), Brannan *et al.* (1975) and Howells (1986) give figures for the incidence of hearing impairment in this group of people ranging from 9.5 per cent to 22.5 per cent. However, the extent to which these figures underestimated the problem is demonstrated by a very comprehensive study in Lewisham and North Southwark (Yeates, 1992). When the hearing of a sample of 500 adults with learning difficulties was assessed by a variety of methods, a total of 69 per cent were found to have some degree of hearing loss, 39 per cent being severe enough to require amplification. Yeates' research also illustrates that when testing is carried out by appropriately skilled and experienced personnel, it is possible to obtain a high degree of accuracy in the results. These results have subsequently been supported by other small-scale studies (for example, Williamson and Jenkins, 1995).

The impact of hearing loss

Although the incidence of hearing loss in the population of people with a learning disability is of great importance, a consideration of the impact on individuals, their quality of life and that of their family and carers is equally vital. This can perhaps best be illustrated by telling the stories of two people whose hearing loss had gone unrecognised, and the changes in their lives when, because a specialist service became available, appropriate help and support were provided.

Gordon is in his forties and has no speech, although he uses much gesture. He recently moved into a hostel when the large mental handicap hospital where he had spent most of his life closed. He showed some unexpected abilities in practical activities, but many staff regarded him as 'difficult' and were wary of him because he could be violent and aggressive. Hearing tests had previously been attempted, but their results were inconclusive, with no clear indication of a hearing loss. In 1995, as part of a specially funded study, tests showed that Gordon was, in fact, profoundly deaf and had almost certainly been deaf all his life. He was given a bone conduction hearing aid to enable him to have an awareness of sound through vibration, but most importantly of all, the staff who supported Gordon now had an explanation for why his behaviour was sometimes unpredictable; they could now learn how to communicate with him appropriately and make his world more understandable. Sadly, it is not possible to undo all the harm that Gordon has suffered because his deafness was not recognised, but perhaps the major benefit for him has been a change in attitudes towards him, and a recognition of the many abilities that he has in spite of his dual disability.

David's story is an example of how a deterioration in hearing can go unrecognised, and the effect that this can have. David is 50 years old, has Down's syndrome and lives with his elderly parents. Although David had always been very sociable, he had become increasingly withdrawn, to the extent that he would sometimes just sit alone and cry. He was also communicating less and less by speech. An added complication was that, as with many older people with Down's syndrome, his sight was deteriorating. Hearing tests revealed that he had a severe sensorineural hearing loss, typically associated with ageing, which would benefit from a hearing aid. Although his father was concerned about how David would cope with an aid, once he had tried it David would not be parted from it, and he soon learned to manage it himself. He began to speak again and became more sociable and happier. People commented that David was like 'his old self again'.

These examples raise the question of how many more Davids and Gordons there are whose hearing loss is still undetected and who are not receiving help and support.

Why is there a greater incidence of hearing impairment associated with learning difficulties?

There are more than 30 syndromes associated with learning difficulty that also carry a predisposition to hearing impairment, the most common of which is Down's syndrome. Other causes of learning difficulty linked to hearing loss are infections, either prenatal (rubella and cytomegalovirus) or postnatal (mumps, measles and meningitis), and perinatal factors such as rhesus incompatibility, toxaemia and birth trauma. The following discussion deals with the most widely occurring conditions.

Down's syndrome

The high incidence of hearing problems associated with Down's syndrome has been well established and documented (Davies, 1985). A comprehensive description of hearing impairment in children with Down's syndrome was carried out by Downs in 1980 (Northern and Downs, 1991), in a study of 107 children with Down's syndrome. Seventy-eight per cent were found to have a hearing loss in one or both ears, 54 per cent had conductive loss, 16 per cent sensorineural loss and 8 per cent mixed-type hearing loss.

The hypotonia linked with Down's syndrome, the narrow, floppy external auditory canal, the frequency of upper respiratory tract infections and the high susceptibility to middle ear conditions leading to secretory otitis media (glue ear) all contribute to the problem. In those people without Down's syndrome, untreated glue ear will usually eventually resolve spontaneously and very rarely persists into adult life. However, in people with Down's syndrome, this condition does persist into adulthood, and even where it has been treated surgically by the insertion of grommets, the fluid frequently returns after grommets are removed.

There is also evidence of a high incidence and early onset of presbyacusis (the sensorineural, initially high-frequency hearing loss associated with ageing) in people with Down's syndrome (Buchanan, 1990). If this is combined with the effects of early-onset dementia and possibly unattended vision problems, frustration and confusion are likely to result.

Prematurity and neonatal factors

There are a number of causal factors associated with trauma at or around the time of birth. Premature birth may increase the risk of small bleeds into the cochlea, and of respiratory distress syndrome, while incubator noise has been cited as a possible cause of damage.

A link also exists between anoxia, resultant cerebral palsy and an increased likelihood of mild to moderate sensorineural hearing loss, which is typically more severe in the high frequencies (Northern and Downs, 1991).

Meningitis and rubella

Retrospective studies have found that up to 29 per cent of children who survive bacterial meningitis are left with a hearing loss, (Kaplan *et al.*, 1984). Rubella contracted in the early months of pregnancy can significantly affect the child's hearing and cause abnormalities of the inner, middle and outer ear, as well as the sequelae of prematurity, low birth weight and jaundice associated with congenital rubella (Northern and Downs, 1991).

Cerumen (wax)

People with learning difficulties are considerably more prone to developing excessive and impacted wax than are the general population, this being particularly so for people with Down's syndrome. Crandell and Roeser (1993) found that, over a 12-year period, 28 per cent of their study had excessive or impacted wax in one or both ears compared with 2–6 per cent of people without learning difficulties. They suggested that where the external auditory canal is 80 per cent occluded, a mild conductive loss can result and that complete occlusion may cause a moderate hearing loss of 40–45 decibels. People with limited communication skills will find it difficult to express the deterioration in hearing caused by wax and may become distressed or withdrawn. Impacted wax can also cause 'buzzing' in the affected ear, which may add to the distress. A number of possible reasons for the increased incidence of wax have been suggested, including the size and shape of the external auditory canal, hypotonia and poor chewing movements, either as a result of physical disability or because of a soft diet reducing the need to chew. Whatever the cause, it is an easily treatable condition, which can be largely avoided with proper monitoring.

Tinnitus

Episodes of tinnitus (noise heard in the ear without any external cause) arising spontaneously and lasting for more than 5 minutes were found by Coles (1993) in a large postal survey to have been experienced by 10 per cent of the general population. Four per cent reported tinnitus causing moderate or severe annoyance, 80 per cent of these also reporting sleep disturbance. Although there are no figures for this distressing condition in people with learning difficulties, the increased incidence of hearing problems, particularly impacted wax and serous otitis media, which are known to be linked with tinnitus, would lead to the expectation that a significant number of people with learning difficulties could be affected by tinnitus and that tinnitus could conceivably be associated with problem behaviour. This is an area that would benefit from further research.

So far, this chapter has been concerned with establishing and describing the nature and extent of the coexistence of learning difficulties and hearing impairment. The issues arising, in particular the implications for providing an effective service, can be divided into two main areas: first, identification and diagnosis, and second, appropriate treatment, management and on-going support. These will be explored in the next sections.

Identification and diagnosis

Awareness of the problem

Until recently, it was widely accepted that the incidence of hearing impairment in people with learning difficulties was in the region of 10–20 per cent. However, the Lewisham and North Southwark study (Yeates, 1992) produced a very much higher figure and raised the awareness of the potential extent of the problem. For some staff working in services for people with learning difficulties, there was already a concern that the number of people with an identified hearing loss did not even reach the earlier estimates of 10–20 per cent, let alone the figures in excess of 50 per cent found in Lewisham and North Southwark.

Although it is difficult to find documentary support for this, a study by the Royal College of General Practitioners (Howells, 1986) did find evidence that a number of conditions, including hearing impairment, went unrecognised and unmanaged. Confirmation of this comes in a study by Shearman (1994), in which only two out of a sample of 100 people attending a social services day centre in an area with no specialist hearing impairment and learning disability service had had their hearing tested within the previous 2 years. When this group of people was followed up and given hearing tests, 47 per cent had some degree of hearing loss, 5 per cent had a possible hearing impairment, and 2 per cent gave inconsistent responses to testing (Williamson and Jenkins, 1995).

In order to improve the level of identification, there needs to be a wider awareness of the extent of the problem and how it can be recognised. People who have learning difficulties, their families and carers, other professionals, including general practitioners (GPs), and specialist staff should have information and training so that they can recognise the signs of hearing loss and know how to obtain access to hearing tests and appropriate treatment and advice. They may also need to know, and possibly to convince others, that the time, effort and financial costs involved are worthwhile, with resulting improvements in quality of life for the individual and, in many cases, for their families too. There is the additional potential for reducing the long-term costs to services of misdiagnosis, treatment and increased dependency. It is, however, important to be aware that someone's hearing status can change. The fact that hearing has been tested in the past and found to be normal does not rule out the possibility of a future hearing problem.

Testing to obtain accurate results

Even when the possibility of a hearing loss is acknowledged and access to testing is available, there remains the problem of accurately determining the extent and nature of any hearing loss, especially when the learning difficulties are severe or profound, or other problems (visual, physical or behavioural) are also present. Some of these difficulties have been discussed earlier in the chapter, but, as Yeates' (1992) study demonstrates, many of these problems can be overcome with effort and experience.

Although pure tone audiometry involves the person being tested wearing earphones and making a deliberate response to a sound, where someone is not able to give this level of cooperation, it is possible to use free field audiometry and to observe their reactions to a range of frequencies and volume. The McCormick Speech Test can be useful for those with some verbal understanding. Tympanometry, in which a small probe put into the ear provides confirmation of conductive deafness, together with testing of the acoustic reflex, requires minimal cooperation, although a few people will not tolerate this procedure. The brainstem evoked response test can be performed without cooperation, but as it may require the use of light anaesthesia, there are ethical issues when someone is not able to give informed consent (Yeates, 1992).

However, in addition to the method used, two very important factors that influence the validity of the testing are the experience of the tester and the preparation prior to the test. The majority of audiology staff, no matter how experienced they are at testing hearing and how sympathetic they may be to people with learning difficulties, have received no specific training or information on the special needs of this group of people. If they are working in a busy hospital clinic, they will almost certainly have time constraints for each individual tested. Ear, nose and throat consultants, however willing to help, may not know how to gain the cooperation of the patient, who may be frightened or disturbed in unfamiliar surroundings.

There are at least three ways in which careful preparation can assist in making the results of testing more meaningful. The first is simply ensuring that the individual's ears have been checked (by a GP or other competent professional) for excessive wax and treated if necessary. Not only does impacted wax have an effect on hearing acuity, but it also presents great difficulty in carrying out a hearing test. Out of 39 tests attempted with people in institutional care in one district between 1989 and 1990, 43.6 per cent of clients had an excessive amount of wax in one or both of their ears, and audiological testing could not therefore be attempted.

Second, it is now accepted that people with severe learning difficulties can acquire new skills with appropriate teaching, and it has become apparent that time spent 'conditioning' or training people to cooperate with hearing tests can lead to a significantly improved accuracy of results. For many people, only two or three short training sessions are necessary to achieve an adequate level of performance (Shearman, 1994).

Third, a detailed history, or profile of the individual, compiled beforehand, can be very helpful, both to the tester and to the individual and his or her family. This history should contain not only details of any previous illness, especially ear infections, but also details of medication as there has been speculation that some combinations of medication can suppress the acoustic reflex

(Niswander and Helfner, 1988), and some drugs prescribed for epilepsy can cause drowsiness. Any visual problems should be noted, together with some information about individuals, their likes and dislikes, and how they are likely to respond to the testing. Gathering the information for this profile can also be used as an opportunity for counselling and for reassuring clients and their families with regard to the test.

Treatment, management and support

Audiological assessment can only be one step in a process to enable the successful therapeutic rehabilitation of a hearing impairment to take place. Once diagnosed, the hearing loss needs to be treated in a holistic way, having regard to the individual's needs and wishes across all areas of his or her life, with appropriate and on-going support available.

Hearing aids

The provision of a hearing aid alone is rarely the solution to the problem. Research carried out by Williams (1993) found that, of people with learning difficulties who had been fitted with an aid, only 66 per cent were using them regularly. Many people working in services would consider this to be a better than average rate, as Shearman found in her comparison of services in two similar NHS Trusts, one with a specialist service for people with learning difficulties and hearing impairment, and one without (Shearman, 1994). In her study, of 10 people interviewed in the non-specialist service area, only two wore their aids regularly. It can be counter-productive to provide aids that are then not used, as providers may decide that it is a waste of resources, and families and direct care staff may feel that there is no point in going through the process of referral and testing if no benefit accrues for the individual.

This raises the question of why so many aids are not used. There is not one simple answer to this question but a number of contributory factors, some of them interdependent. In some cases, the aids provided are not the most suitable for the particular type of hearing loss or fail to take into account other problems that the individual may have. This may be because the information gained from the hearing test was not sufficiently detailed or accurate to enable a properly informed decision to be made, or it may be that the most appropriate types of aid, or adaptations to aids, are not provided by the NHS. Many people with learning difficulties are dependent on state benefits and cannot pay privately for an aid. Sometimes an aid is not being used because it is not working and the person with learning difficulties or the carer does not know how to get it repaired. The fault may be as simple as its requiring a fresh battery.

When someone with a learning difficulty is supported by paid staff for most of his or her daily living needs, it is possible that staff changes and poor communication result in support workers not knowing how the aid should be used or even that the person has ever been provided with a hearing aid. Not infrequently, an individual with a learning difficulty will initially reject the hearing aid, either refusing to wear it or removing it after a short time, and this it taken as an indication that the aid is unsuitable. This may be the case, but it is a common misconception that simply providing someone with a hearing aid will bring an immediate benefit. When someone has not heard properly for many years, if ever, suddenly hearing everything at normal volume can be quite a shock, and the aid will almost certainly need to be introduced gradually. Some places or times of the day are particularly noisy, for example lunch or coffee break in the dining room of a large day centre, and wearing an aid at such times may, at least to start with, cause distress. The experience of having an object in the ear can be problematic for some individuals, but this can usually be overcome with a sensitive approach.

Glue ear

There is currently a debate on the most appropriate treatment for serous otitis media in young children, and the pendulum is swinging away from surgical treatment by the insertion of grommets in all but the most persistent cases as research indicates that the condition resolves in time in the majority of cases. There seems to be a dearth of information about how best to treat this condition in adults with learning difficulties, possibly because the extent of the problem has only recently been appreciated. One small study from the Netherlands (Evenhuis et al., 1993), where people with Down's syndrome were given grommets, did not show any measurable benefit from this procedure. However, the number of people involved was very small, and the post-treatment measures were taken only 7 months after surgery. In addition, the mean age of the people involved was over 50 years, an age when it might be thought optimistic to expect a great deal of change to occur.

This is an area in which more research is obviously needed, although there is again the issue of consent to treatment, especially where that treatment is not of proven benefit. Treatment by medication, antibiotics and/or decongestants is usually appropriate and, 'auto-inflation' of the eustachian tube by holding the nose and blowing has proved beneficial for some children, also being non-invasive. Hearing aids have been used with good results.

Modifying the environment

There are a number of environmental measures that, taken alone or together with the provision of a hearing aid, can improve the quality of life for someone who has a hearing loss. Adaptations can be provided, such as fitting an induction loop system so that the hearing aid picks up signals directly from the television, radio or tape player without others having to put up with increased volume. Doorbells and alarm clocks with flashing lights, and amplification for telephones are examples of other devices available. Some measures require no extra resources. It is important that those who are not independently mobile sit where they can easily see what is happening and will not be taken by surprise if people suddenly appear. Simply ensuring that the light is good enough for people to read lips or facial expressions, and that there is not too much extraneous noise, can bring many benefits. All of this of course emphasises the importance of providing adequate information and training for families and carers when a hearing loss is diagnosed.

Ongoing management and support

The research information available, together with evidence from staff and families, demonstrates clearly that ongoing support is necessary for people with learning difficulties, even when the loss has been identified, if they are to gain any improvement in their quality of life. Where this support is available, benefits can be seen in terms of increased independence. A significant number of people have learned to use their hearing aids with minimal support, with a resulting growth in confidence and self-esteem.

Even where this is not possible, the presence of support can influence whether an aid is worn (or whether it is left sitting in a drawer) and whether other beneficial changes occur, such as other people learning how they can communicate meaningfully with someone who has a hearing loss. It is vital that this support is maintained in the long term in order to deal with difficulties as they arise and to monitor and review any changes in hearing status. There is also the need for a responsible person with appropriate skills and experience to coordinate the support required, also ensuring that everybody involved is kept informed and has the knowledge and training to provide high-quality support for people with learning difficulties and hearing impairment.

Having highlighted the needs of people who experience both learning difficulties and hearing impairment, how can effective services to meet these needs be provided?

Services to meet the needs of people with learning difficulties and hearing impairment

How should services be provided – generic or specialist?

Almost without exception, services for people with learning difficulties base their philosophies on John O'Brien's five accomplishments (O'Brien and Tyne, 1981). The accomplishments of 'community presence' and 'participation', when applied to health care in the context of 'an ordinary life', are often seen as indicating that people with learning difficulties should use generic rather than specialist health services. Specialist services can be regarded as another form of segregation, with all the negative connotations associated with labelling. However, it can be argued that emphasis on using generic services does in fact restrict the rights of people with learning difficulties to have their health needs properly addressed. It is not unreasonable to infer from evidence already presented in this chapter that generic services have so far singularly failed to meet the special needs of this group.

This discussion should, of course, be seen in the context of poor service provision of all kinds for people with a learning difficulty in the recent past. In many areas, access to mainstream audiology services was severely restricted, if not totally blocked, for a number of reasons. In some instances, this was simply because of a lack of awareness of either the needs themselves or anything that could be done to provide effective treatment. In other cases, it was more a matter of negative attitudes and failure to acknowledge the individual rights of those with learning difficulties. It was felt that resources would be 'wasted' on this group of people. This then becomes a self-fulfilling prophecy, for if people with learning difficulties are not given appropriate support to use generic services, and if these services are not sufficiently flexible to be able to adapt to individual needs, outcomes will be poor – and if outcomes are poor, it may be considered inappropriate (or not cost-effective) to provide treatment. In more recent times, however, there has been a change in attitudes, with a growing awareness of the need to provide equal access to all, even though there may be a lack of knowledge of the best way to do this and a lack of the necessary resources.

In a 1994 study comparing two similar areas, one with a specialist hearing therapy and audiological service and one using a non-specialist, hospital-based audiological service, Shearman found that, with the specialist service, a much larger number of people with learning difficulties had had hearing tests, and the results and recommendations from the tests were more informative. Where hearing aids had been supplied, there was a higher use of aids and greater satisfaction with support provided in the area with the specialist service. There are, of course, things that a specialist service cannot provide economically, such as specialised and expensive items of equipment for testing for brainstem evoked responses, or facilities and skills for surgical intervention.

But does a service have to be either specialist or generic? *The Health of the Nation: A Strategy for People with Learning Disabilities*, (DoH, 1995) recommended that those who commission health services specify in their contracts 'Health services which enable people with learning disabilities to use health services available to everyone else; and specialist health services where these are necessary' (p. 38). The document also stated that, in addition to enabling people with learning difficulties to 'obtain access to all the community resources available to others, with support' (p. 11), elements of health surveillance programmes should also concentrate on 'Detecting additional needs and referring for specialist advice (for example... sight and hearing problems)' (p. 15).

In the few areas of the country, such as Lewisham and North Southwark, and Derbyshire, where there are good models of service provision, this is what is happening. People who are able to make use of generic services are supported to do so, but a specialist service is available for those with greater and more complex needs.

This specialist service will also link into the mainstream service to ensure an efficient use of resources.

What should services provide?

It is not enough simply to provide access to audiology services for people with learning difficulties. The very high incidence of hearing problems that has recently emerged indicates that a more proactive approach is required, with regular screening, especially for those at greatest risk, such as those with Down's syndrome and profound and multiple disabilities. The most important factor in effective service delivery, however, is probably the presence of staff with skill and experience.

Another important ingredient of an effective service is the availability of information in an easily accessible form for people with learning difficulties, their families and the staff who support them. Written material should use simple language, possibly supplemented by symbols or pictures, and the use of video- and audio-taped information should be considered. The contents of these should raise the awareness of the likelihood of the co-occurrence of hearing impairment and learning difficulties, as well as of how hearing loss might show itself. There should also be details of how to request a hearing test, and what support and follow-up will be provided if a hearing loss is found. If a hearing aid is provided, there should be instructions for using and maintaining the aid.

Staff training is another way of providing information as it is essential that those in constant contact with people with learning difficulties are able to provide day-to-day support, both in the use and maintenance of hearing aids and in communicating with, and providing an enabling environment for, the people they support.

Who should deliver the service?

Another consideration is the professional qualifications and skills of those actually delivering the service. Which professional group is best equipped to fulfil the key role in coordinating the many and varied strands of an effective service? Hearing therapy is a relatively new profession that aims to provide both technical support and counselling as part of an aural rehabilitation service. Hearing therapists use a holistic approach, based upon respect for the needs and wishes of individual clients. Speech and language therapists, in their initial training, do acquire some knowledge and skills in the management of hearing impairment but they would need additional postgraduate audiology training to coordinate this type of service successfully. Wide experience of working with people with learning difficulties is an essential qualification for this role.

If valid results are to be obtained, training in the special needs of people with learning difficulties is also vital for audiology staff who will be testing hearing whether as part of a specialist service or when dealing with those people who are able to use mainstream services. Good working relationships need to be established with ear, nose and throat consultants and specialists in audiological medicine in order to enable access to facilities that a specialist service alone cannot provide.

Summary

Hearing impairment is an area where there is a major opportunity for health gain and improved quality of life for people with learning difficulties. The current extent of underdiagnosis combined with much ineffective treatment makes this a relatively easy target to achieve.

Checklist for action

- People with learning difficulties who are able to do so should be supported to utilise mainstream audiology services.
- For those who need it, there should be a specialist service coordinated by a key professional, either a hearing therapist or a speech and language therapist with postgraduate training.
- Information to raise awareness of hearing loss and how to access testing should be available in an easily understandable form for people with learning difficulties, their families and their carers.
- Support staff need training about hearing impairment and those who carry out hearing tests need training about the needs of people with learning difficulties.
- A programme of regular screening for hearing loss should be available. Pretest preparation should include the treatment of wax, 'conditioning' and counselling.

- Further research is needed to establish the most effective treatment of conductive hearing loss, particularly for adults with Down's syndrome.
- There should be a flexible policy of providing the most suitable hearing aids to meet individual needs.
- Support should be available to individuals and their carers when a hearing loss has been diagnosed in order for them to gain maximum benefit from their hearing aids and maximum independence in using them. Support for families and carers in adapting the environment is also required.

References

Brannan, A.C., Seligman, C. and Bensberg, G.J. 'The hearing impaired in state institutions for the retarded: prevalance, characteristics and diagnosis.' *American Annals of the Deaf*, **210**(4)(1975): 408–16.
Buchanan, L.H. 'Early onset of presbyacusis in Down's syndrome.' *Scandinavian Audiology Supplement*, **19**(1990): 103–10.
Coles, R. Tinnitus. Paper presented at the International Conference on Hearing Rehabilitation. (Sydney: 14–18 July 1993).
Crandell, C. and Roeser, R. 'Incidence of excessive/impacted cerumen in individuals with mental retardation; a longitudinal investigation'. *American Journal of Mental Retardation*, **97**(5)(1993): 568–74.
Davies, B. 'Hearing problems', in Lane D. and Stratford B. (eds) *Current Approaches to Down's Syndrome*. (London: Cassell, 1985, pp. 85–102).
Department of Health. *The Health of the Nation: A Strategy for People with Learning Disabilities*. (London: HMSO, 1995).
Evenhuis, H.M., Van Lier, P.A., Hakker, A.A., Roerdinkholder, W.H.M. and De Bruin, W.C.M. 'Effects of treatment of hearing loss in middle-aged persons with Down's syndrome: a pilot study.' *International Journal of Disability, Development and Education*. **40**(2)(1993): 159–62.
Howells, G. 'Are the medical needs of mentally handicapped adults being met?' *Journal of the Royal College of General Practioners*, **33**(1986): 449–53.
Kaplan, S.L., Catlin, F., Weaver, T. and Feigin, R.D. 'Onset of hearing loss in children with bacterial meningitis.' *Paediatrics*, **73**(1984): 575–9.
Lloyd, L. and Reid, M.J. 'The incidence of hearing impairment in an institutionalised mentally retarded population.' *American Journal of Mental Deficiency*, **71**(5)(1967): 746–63.
Niswander, P.S. and Helfner, M. 'Observations on the acoustic reflex threshold in institutionalised retarded adults taking mellaril and/or thorazine.' *Ear and Hearing*, **9**(1)(1988): 9–14.
Northern, J.L. and Downs, M. *Hearing in Children*. (Baltimore: Williams & Wilkins, 1991).
O'Brien, J. and Tyne, A. *The Principle of Normalisation: A Foundation for Effective Services*. (London: Campaign for Mentally Handicapped People, 1981).

Shearman, S.J. Do clients with a learning disability benefit from a specialist hearing therapy and audiology service? Unpublished MSc Research Study. (Portsmouth: University of Portsmouth, 1994).

Stewart, L.G. 'Hearing impaired/developmentally disabled persons in the United States: definitions, causes, effects and prevalence estimates.' *American Annals of the Deaf*, **123**(1978): 488–95.

Williams, C. *Hearing Impairment and Learning Disability: Double Jeopardy.* Paper presented at the Annual Conference of the British Institute of Learning Disabilities. (Torquay: September 1993).

Williamson, S. and Jenkins, C. Hearing impairment in adults with a learning disability. Unpublished research study. (Swindon: East Wiltshire Healthcare NHS Trust, 1995).

Yeates, S. 'Have they got a hearing loss?' *Mental Handicap*, December (1992): 126–33.

9

MANAGEMENT OF SLEEP DISORDERS IN CHILDREN WITH LEARNING DIFFICULTIES

Rebecca Stores, Luci Wiggs and Gregory Stores

Sleep is a fundamental human need, essential for promoting healthy physical growth and development. Children's sleep problems are common and can have serious effects on both the child and other members of the family. Such problems are even more prevalent in children with learning difficulties and are frequently referred to by parents as a cause of considerable stress. This chapter will give a brief introduction to the topic of sleep problems and their effects on both the child and the family.

Prevalence of sleep problems

The rate of sleep disturbance in children in the general population is high, even for the more severe and persistently occurring disturbances (for example, in 25 per cent of pre-school children, 43 per cent aged 8–10 years and 33 per cent of adolescents). Particularly common are problems of settling to sleep and waking in the night. Settling problems have been reported in 22 per cent of 9-month-old babies, 15–20 per cent of 1–2-year-olds and 16–18 per cent of 3-year-olds. Night waking is even more common, affecting 42 per cent of children aged 9 months, 20–26 per cent of 1–2-year-olds, 14–22 per cent of 3-year-olds and even 10 per cent of those aged 4.5 years.

There have been only a limited number of studies looking at the prevalence and effects of sleep disorders in children with learning difficulties, most having focused on problems of sleeplessness (settling, night waking and early waking difficulties). The evidence suggests that the prevalence of these problems is alarmingly high in this population, even into late adolescence. Table 9.1 shows the main findings from previous studies.

Table 9.1 Sleep disturbance in studies of
children with learning difficulties

Study	Number of children	Age (years)	Sleep problem	Percentage
Pahl and Quine (1984)	200	Up to 18	Settling problems	51
			Night waking problems	67
Bartlett *et al.* (1985)	214	Up to 16	Settling problems	56
			Night waking problems	56
			Going to bed	53
Clements *et al.* (1986)	155	Up to 15	Sleep problems	34

Sleep problems are not only common in children with learning difficulties, but also exceedingly persistent. Quine (1991) performed a 3-year follow-up of the subjects in an earlier study and found that 48 per cent of the children with settling problems still presented with problems, as did 66 per cent of the children with night waking problems. Twenty-one per cent of children had developed sleep problems that had not been present 3 years previously.

The widespread and persistent nature of sleep problems in children and adolescents with learning difficulties is particularly worrying in view of the fact that childhood sleep problems have been seen to be associated with a number of undesirable factors. The existence of these negative associations highlights the need for sleep problems to be diagnosed and for intervention to begin as soon as possible, especially as successful intervention has been seen to result in improvement of many of the associated variables.

The importance of sleep disruption for learning and behaviour in children with learning difficulties

Sleep problems are often part of a more general behaviour disturbance in the child. About three times the usual rate of daytime behaviour problems are seen in children with sleep problems. Tantrums and food fads are particularly common.

Children with learning difficulties and sleep problems have also been reported to have more daytime behaviour problems than those without sleep problems. Quine (1991) found that the parents of children with sleep problems reported higher levels of behaviour

problems and were more likely to describe their child as very difficult to manage, unable to be left unsupervised and in need of more
attention. Educational levels, self-help abilities and incontinence
were all lower among the children with sleep problems, but the
greatest difference between those with and those without sleep
problems was seen in the area of communication skills: about a
third of children with sleep problems had a poor use and understanding of communication, compared with only a tenth of the non-
sleep problem group. Epilepsy was also associated, suggesting
neurological impairment, or nocturnal seizures, as a possible cause
of sleep problems.

In addition to these disorders of sleeplessness, sleep-related
breathing disorders have also been shown to be linked to various
adverse effects. The majority of research on this topic has focused
on individuals in the general population. In children, daytime
symptoms include irritability, hyperactivity, aggression, learning
problems, developmental delay and reduced attention and concentration skills. It is probable that the same consequences will occur in
children with learning difficulties and may be misinterpreted as
part of the learning disabled condition. Such consequences may
significantly add to the degree of disability already experienced.

There are a number of ways in which a child's sleep problem
could be contributing to these learning and behaviour difficulties.
First, reduced sleep duration or continuity has been seen to result in
changes in behaviour including regressive behaviour, euphoria,
aggression, antisocial behaviour, irritability and brief psychotic
states. Cognitive changes have also been apparent: concentration,
reaction time and even creative thought have been seen to be
impaired. The length of the period for which one has to concentrate
seems to be of primary importance (subjects performing less well
over a long period), indicating that situations requiring sustained
attention (for example, lessons at school) may be those on which
sleep disruption is likely to have most negative effect (Bonnet, 1994).

Second, the most consistent finding is, not surprisingly, that
sleep-deprived humans are sleepy. This occurs both after a night of
restricted sleep duration or following sleep fragmented by brief
arousals that may not necessarily reduce total sleep duration. Brief
lapses into sleep for a few seconds (microsleeps) have been seen to
increase in number as the length of deprivation increases. These
lapses may have significant consequences for performance: sleepy
children may not simply be tired but may actually be asleep at
times when they are supposed to be learning. It is of course not

only the children themselves who suffer from disturbed sleep; the carers of children with sleep problems will also have disturbed sleep and may themselves be too sleepy to teach appropriate behaviour to their child or to correct inappropriate behaviour should it occur.

Of note is that children may take longer than adults to recover from sleep disruption. Although children have been seen to be significantly sleepy during the day following sleep restriction, they do not show the usual rebound sleep on the recovery night when they are allowed to sleep. The effects of accumulated sleep loss in children need investigation.

Third, sleeping medication (usually antihistamines or chloral hydrate) can further contribute to daytime drowsiness.

Associations between sleep problems and parenting, partnerships and family life

It is difficult to unravel the cause and effect relationships of the interactions between a child, its carer and its environment. However, a number of family factors are clearly associated with having a child with a sleep problem.

Mothers of children in the general population with sleep problems have received the greatest amount of attention in the research literature, but other family members have been investigated, including the siblings of children with sleep problems (who were often reported by parents to have had sleep problems in the past) and fathers (who were more likely to be described by mothers as being unsupportive and difficult to confide in). In mothers, a high incidence of depression, anxiety and alcohol dependency have been identified. Marital difficulties are also more common. Differences have been noted in the care taking of mothers of children with and without sleep problems: those with children with sleep problems are more likely to be ambivalent towards the child. Overstimulation and overresponsiveness by the parents, which may interfere with a child's ability to develop its own self-regulation, has also been noted to be related to nocturnal waking and crying.

Similar associations (albeit usually more marked) have been found in the mothers of children with learning difficulties and sleep problems, for example increased stress, irritability, poorer marital relationships and more negative views of their spouses, their child and themselves (Quine, 1992). The severity of the sleep problem is also important. The more severe the sleep problem, the more the parents consider their child to have an adverse impact on family life and daily functioning (issues not directly related to sleep). As the presence of a learning-disabled child in these families may be expected to cause more stress anyway, the additional problem of sleep difficulties appears to compound their troubles and increase the burden of care.

That the effects of sleep problems on the family unit can be very serious is suggested by the preliminary study by Chavin and Tinson (1980), who interviewed the parents of children aged 8–36 months; 37 per cent felt that the sleep problem had caused serious arguments, 8 per cent admitted severely abusing their child, and 2 per cent attributed the break up of their marriage directly to the child's sleep problem. It has been suggested that poor sleep can lead to parental violence because the poor sleep pattern is often one of a multitude of other associated problems. Encouragingly, there is good evidence that successful behavioural treatments for child sleep problems results in improved child behaviour, parent–child relationships and mental state of the parents (Quine, 1992).

Types of sleep disorder in children with learning difficulties

Virtually all childhood sleep disorders that occur in the general population can occur in children with learning difficulties: there are no sleep disorders that are specific to such children. However, as will be described later, individuals with some forms of learning difficulty are particularly prone to developing specific sleep disorders.

A wide range of childhood sleep disorders exist (Diagnostic Classification Steering Committee, 1997). Their onset and maintenance can have a physical cause, a psychological cause or both. Some, such as infantile colic, are more likely to occur at certain ages, whereas others may appear during childhood and then persist throughout most of the individual's life.

In the following sections, childhood sleep disorders are described under the following headings: disorders associated with sleeplessness, disorders associated with excessive daytime sleepiness, circadian rhythm disorders and night-time attacks (parasomnias).

Sleeplessness

Problems associated with sleeplessness are among the most common sleep problems in children with learning difficulties. They include difficulty in settling the child to sleep, repeated night-time waking with demands for parental attention, early morning waking and persistent short duration sleep.

Possible factors that bring about these disorders are numerous and may vary from child to child. In some cases, a child may have challenging behaviour, the night-time disturbances being just another feature of the problem. In other cases, the presence of a physical or medical disorder such as otitis media or another painful condition may lead to disturbed sleep.

More commonly, the settling and night waking problems develop as a result of the children never having learnt to fall asleep without their parents present. Thus, when they awaken during the night, they are unable to resettle themselves and demand their parents' attention. Such problems are known as 'sleep association disorders'.

In the pre-school or school-aged child, parents' inability or unwillingness to establish and consistently enforce rules for going to bed or staying in bed during the night can lead to irregular sleep patterns and night-time disturbances. These problems are known as 'limit setting disorders'.

In older children, bad sleeping habits and inadequate sleep hygiene may lead to sleeping difficulties. Emotional upset, stress and worry may also cause sleep disruption, as will the existence of any additional psychiatric conditions such as anxiety or depression.

Excessive daytime sleepiness

Excessive daytime sleepiness can have considerable psychological and social effects on any individual. It is rarely seen as a medical problem by parents or professionals, and symptoms may be misinterpreted as laziness, disinterest or lack of motivation. In addition, sleepiness in children can manifest itself quite differently from sleepiness in adults, causing a variety of undesirable behaviours such as irritability, aggression, poor concentration and attention, and hyperactivity. Such problems may be attributed to causes other than sleeplessness, especially in children with learning difficulties.

Excessive daytime sleepiness may be the result of insufficient sleep caused by any of the disorders of sleeplessness described earlier or it may be the result of more specific sleep disorders that have an intrinsic, physical origin. One such disorder is described below.

Obstructive sleep apnoea is a problem that occurs in approximately 2 per cent of the adult and child general population. It is, however, being increasingly recognised at a much higher rate in individuals with a range of specific learning difficulties (described below).

It is a problem of disordered breathing during sleep and occurs as a result of the upper airway becoming blocked during sleep. The blockage is usually caused by muscle hypotonia and narrowing of the upper airway. Each time this occurs, breathing stops for a time and the individual is then woken up by the struggle to breathe. These interruptions in breathing (apnoeas) may occur hundreds of times during the night, causing considerable sleep disruption.

Nocturnal features include loud snoring, restless sleep, sleeping with the neck extended, other unusual sleeping positions, coughing and choking, observed apnoeas, excessive sweating and bedwetting. Daytime consequences include excessive sleepiness, behaviour and personality changes, and impaired concentration and attention. There is evidence to suggest that this problem is underrecognised in the general population and probably more so in individuals with learning difficulties.

Circadian rhythm sleep disorders

These sleep disorders occur when there is a shift in the individuals' sleep phase so that they are unable to sleep at a socially acceptable time. Because they are rarely able to obtain the amount of sleep they require, they experience symptoms of sleeplessness or excessive daytime sleepiness. Delayed sleep phase syndrome is one of the most common sleep–wake rhythm disorders. In this, the individual is physiologically unable to fall asleep until the early hours of the morning and, if given the chance, does not wake up until the afternoon. As these individuals usually have to get up for school or work before their sleep requirements have been met, they are sleepy during the day. Advanced sleep phase syndrome is also possible, the individual falling asleep in the early evening and then wakening in the early hours of the morning. This is, however, generally less common.

In severely learning disabled children (especially those with visual defects), the sleep–wake cycle may be very irregular or other than 24 hours in duration because the child has not been able to properly appreciate the difference between night and day, and associated activities.

Night-time attacks

There are a range of unusual behaviours that occur during sleep or are made worse by sleep, otherwise being known as the parasomnias. Different parasomnias are linked to different stages of sleep and therefore occur at different times during the night. They are more common in childhood and adolescence, and may result in significant distress to the child and/or other family members. The most commonly occurring parasomnias are outlined in Table 9.2.

Table 9.2 Parasomnias and their usual timing during sleep

Parasomnia	Usual timing
Rhythmic movement disorders	Sleep onset
Arousal disorders	First third of the night
Nightmares	Last third of the night
Bed wetting	Any time of the night

Rhythmic movement disorders usually occur at the onset of sleep but also when the child wakes during the night and tries to return to sleep. They include head banging, head rolling and body rocking. These disorders are usually interpreted as a soothing rhythmical activity that aids the onset of sleep. In most cases, no treatment is necessary, parents can be reassured, and the child outgrows the behaviour. However, where there is a risk of injury, protective measures or behavioural techniques are appropriate. Similar rhythmic movements during the day are usually indicative of more serious psychological disturbance, in which case treatment of the underlying problem is necessary.

Arousal disorders are parasomnias that happen during the deeper stages of sleep. They are known as arousal disorders because their occurrence is associated with a partial arousal from these sleep stages to a lighter stage of sleep (but without actual waking during the episode). They are most common during the first third of the night, when deep sleep is most abundant. During these partial arousals, the individual remains asleep during the episode, although older children, adolescents and adults may wake briefly at the end. They include confusional arousals (mainly in young children), sleep walking and sleep/night terrors.

During confusional arousals, the child usually moans or fumbles in a confused manner, cries or even screams and may thrash or kick for perhaps 15 minutes or longer. Treatment is typically unnecessary as the episodes stop spontaneously with time, but explanation and reassurance for the parents is often required.

Sleep walking episodes can range from wandering aimlessly to agitated attempts to 'escape'. Urination in inappropriate places can also occur. The episode usually terminates spontaneously, the individual returning to bed and continuing to sleep. He or she will usually have no memory of the event the next morning. Sleep walking is most prevalent between the ages of 4 and 8 years. The environment needs to be made safe to avoid injury during sleep walking episodes.

Sleep (or night) terrors are characterised by a sudden arousal, with a piercing scream or cry and a terrified expression. The child usually sits up in bed with staring eyes, a very rapid pulse and profuse sweating. More dramatic episodes can involve running about as if trying to escape from something. The episode may last from one to several minutes before it terminates spontaneously and the individual returns to sleep. As in other arousal disorders, parents are encouraged not to wake the individual during an episode because if awoken, the child is likely to become confused and frightened. It is best to let the event take its natural course.

Nightmares are frightening dreams that usually wake the individual. They usually occur during the last third of the night when dreaming sleep (rapid eye movement or REM sleep) is most likely to occur. They may be caused by frightening experiences including television programmes, bedtime stories or more serious psychological trauma. They are more common in childhood than adulthood.

Nightmares and night/sleep terrors are sometimes confused with each other, but a number of factors differentiate the two. In the case of nightmares, parents are usually able to comfort the child. This is not the case with night terrors, in which the individual is not awake during the episode (although older children may wake at the end of it) and may well resist any attempts at comfort. In addition, nightmares usually occur during the second half of the night when REM sleep is most abundant, whereas night/sleep terrors tend to occur towards the beginning of the night.

Bed wetting is a common problem in childhood. It can occur in all stages of sleep. It may be the result of an underlying physical abnormality, for example a urinary tract infection, diabetes, epilepsy or sleep apnoea, in which case treatment of the underlying disorder should resolve the problem. In some cases, it may have an emotional basis. Behavioural techniques are generally the preferred form of treatment.

There are a number of other parasomnias that do not occur during any particular sleep stage. The most common are teeth grinding and sleep talking.

It is important not to confuse the above sleep disorders with nocturnal epileptic attacks or seizures as seizures need a very different approach regarding the investigation of their cause and their treatment. Seizures that are not convulsive in type may well be thought to be nightmares or arousal disorders, and at times the opposite mistake occurs (Stores, 1991). Important clues to the epileptic nature of the attack include a tendency to occur at any time of the night (although there are definite exceptions to this rule) and the occurrence of similar attacks in wakefulness during the day. EEG recordings during the episodes are appropriate when the diagnosis is in doubt.

Sleep disorders in specific forms of learning difficulty

Some specific forms of learning difficulty are particularly associated with certain sleep problems, usually because of certain characteristic physical features associated with the condition. Individuals with Down's syndrome, craniofacial syndromes and the mucopolysaccharidoses have all been shown to be at particular risk of obstructive sleep apnoea. Daytime sleepiness is also a common feature of Prader–Willi syndrome. Sleep studies have indicated that some of these cases have obstructive sleep apnoea, but others do not. Some children with cerebral palsy also have sleep-related breathing problems. Sleep disruption caused by epilepsy seems to be particularly likely in children with cerebral palsy and those with tuberous sclerosis.

Management of sleep disorders

Behavioural and cognitive approaches

Behavioural techniques have been shown to be very effective in the management of childhood sleeplessness and sleep–wake cycle disorders in children with severe learning difficulties (Quine, 1992). Such techniques aim to change the way in which parents react and deal with the problem. A programme of change is agreed between parents and health professional, parents keeping a diary before, during and after the implementation of the various techniques. Techniques that have been used successfully include systematic ignoring, positive reinforcement, shaping/graded approaches and antecedent conditioning.

In addition, many parents benefit from being taught basic principles of 'sleep hygiene'. This term refers to general advice that may help to promote good sleeping patterns; the specific principles are outlined in Table 9.3. Poor sleep hygiene is a common cause of sleep problems, and many such problems can be resolved, or at least mitigated, by adhering to these basic principles.

Medication

Medication for sleep disorders is among that most commonly prescribed in clinical practice. At any age, the long-term use of benzodiazepine hypnotics is discouraged because of problems of dependence and hangover effects. They are usually reserved for short-term use if really necessary. In young children, antihistamine or chloral drugs are often prescribed even though there is no good evidence of their effectiveness when used for long periods.

Melatonin has been used recently in the treatment of the sleep–wake cycle disorders. This is a naturally occurring hormone released from the pituitary gland during sleep that works by regulating the sleep–wake cycle. It has been reported to be of use in children with severe learning difficulties, but further careful evaluation is needed.

Table 9.3   General advice for improving children's sleep hygiene

- The sleeping environment should be physically conducive to sleep, that is quiet, dark, avoiding extremes of temperature and without disturbance from other people, and the bed should be comfortable

- The sleeping environment should be familiar, comforting and relaxing, being associated with sleep rather than play or entertainment

- The bedroom should not be a place of punishment or have other negative associations

- There should be a consistent evening and bedtime routine ending with the child being relaxed and ready for sleep

- Bedtime and waking-up time should be consistent, including weekends and holidays (within reason)

- The child should be put to bed when tired

- Children should learn to fall asleep on their own without their parents being present

- A pattern confining feeding to daytime and sleeping to night should be promoted early in development and maintained

- Hunger at bedtime should be avoided, but excessive fluids at bedtime or during the night, as well as heavy meals later at night, should be avoided

- Parents should avoid reinforcing settling and waking problems by giving in to demands for drinks, food, more stories and so on in an attempt to avoid confrontation

- Naps in young children should not be too early or late in the day, or be too many or too few in number

- Boisterous play or other arousing activities (including frightening videos or stories) should be avoided in the hour or so before bedtime

- Stimulant-containing drinks (cola, coffee, chocolate and tea) should be avoided for several hours before going to bed, and excessive amounts avoided during the day.

Other physical treatments

There are a range of other physical treatments that are used mainly in the management of obstructive sleep apnoea. These include various surgical interventions, such as the removal of the tonsils and adenoids. For adults in the general population, the most common form of treatment is continuous positive airway pressure (CPAP). This treatment involves the individual wearing a mask that is placed over the nose and mouth during sleep through which air is pumped continuously to keep the airway open. Experience of its use in children is limited.

Problems with current services

The current services in the UK for these problems are limited. Research suggests that the wide range of sleep problems, particularly in children with learning difficulties, often goes underrecognised, inaccurately diagnosed and consequently undermanaged (Wiggs and Stores, 1996a). One of the most important reasons for this shortfall appears to be the lack of training in this area given to health professionals, including doctors and psychologists (Wiggs and Stores, 1996b).

A further problem is that only a handful of specialised sleep clinics exist. As with the research in this area, services for children in the general population lag behind those for adults, and individuals with learning difficulties fare even less well than other sections of the population.

Solutions and recommendations

To ensure that sleep problems are recognised quickly, investigated, diagnosed accurately and managed properly, the amount of *professional training* in this area needs to be increased. It is difficult to include all the pertinent and important components in training courses, but there are a number of ways in which the teaching of, and interest in, sleep-related topics can be encouraged (see Wiggs and Stores, 1996b) without compromising other aspects of training. Such training is necessary for a range of professionals, including general practitioners, paediatricians, psychiatrists, psychologists, health visitors and others involved in the daily care of children with learning difficulties (for example, respite carers). Professionals need to be made aware of the range of potentially successful treatment possibilities for sleep problems in children with learning difficulties.

The increased existence of *specialised sleep clinics* would assist in the process of recognition: carers would be encouraged to present problems, and health professionals to enquire about them, if a place of referral existed where help could be sought. It is equally important that a *multidisciplinary approach* to the diagnosis and management of sleep disorders in these children is incorporated into such a system. Sleep patterns need to be enquired about regularly and routinely so that early intervention is possible. They should preferably not be dealt with in isolation but by a team of professionals responsible for other aspects of a child's care, many of which may interact with sleep problems and issues of management (for example, epilepsy, health problems and behaviour problems).

For many of the common sleep problems of settling and night waking, behavioural treatments are the most appropriate, so the *role of carers* in intervention needs to be stressed. Family preferences and circumstances need to be considered by someone who has a good knowledge of the family as a unit and who can support the carers during any intervention. Health visitors and other community workers with whom the family has regular contact may be best placed to fill this role.

Checklist for action

- Children with learning difficulties should have the same access rights to all general health services involved in the management of sleep disorders as are granted to children in the general population.
- Increased training on the diagnosis and management of sleep problems is vital for health professionals involved in the care of children with learning difficulties.
- It is essential that more research is conducted in order to understand the pattern of sleep problems in specific types of learning difficulty more fully, so that appropriate screening and treatment methods can be developed and assessed. In particular, the possibility of prevention needs investigation.
- There is an urgent need for increased support and advice for the carers of children with learning difficulties who have a sleep problem.
- A coordinated multidisciplinary approach to the diagnosis and management of sleep problems in children with learning difficulties is required.
- Individual screening programmes should be developed for the various forms of learning difficulty, especially those in which certain sleep problems are more likely to occur.

References

Bartlett, L.B., Rooney, V. and Spedding, S. 'Nocturnal difficulties in a population of mentally handicapped children.' *British Journal of Mental Subnormality*, **31**(1985): 54–9.

Bonnet, M.H. 'Sleep deprivation', in Kryger, M.H., Roth, T. and Dement, W.C. (eds) *Principles and Practice of Sleep Medicine* (2nd edn). (Philadelphia : WB Saunders, 1994, pp. 50–67).

Chavin, W. and Tinson, S. 'Children with sleep difficulties.' *Health Visitor*, **53**(1980): 477–80.

Clements, J., Wing, L. and Dunn, G. 'Sleep problems in handicapped children: a preliminary study.' *Journal of Child Psychology and Psychiatry*, **27**(1986): 399–407.

Diagnostic Classification Steering Committee. *The International Classification of Sleep Disorders: Diagnostic and Coding Manual.* (Rochester, MN: American Sleep Disorder Association, 1997, rev. edn).

Pahl, J. and Quine, L. *Families with Mentally Handicapped Children: A Study of Stress and of Service Response.* (Canterbury: Health Services Research Unit, University of Kent at Canterbury, 1984).

Quine, L. 'Sleep problems in children with severe mental handicap.' *Journal of Mental Deficiency Research*, **35**(1991): 269–90.

Quine, L. 'Helping parents to manage children's sleep disturbance. An intervention trial using health professionals', in Gibbons J. (ed.) *The Children Act 1989 and Family Support: Principles into Practice.* (London: HMSO, 1992, pp. 101–41).

Stores, G. 'Confusions concerning sleep disorders and the epilepsies in children and adolescents.' *British Journal of Psychiatry*, **158**(1991): 1–7.

Wiggs, L. and Stores, G. 'Sleep problems in children with severe learning disabilities: what help is being provided?' *Journal of Applied Research in Intellectual Disability*, **9**(1996a): 160–5.

Wiggs, L. and Stores, R. 'Sleep education in undergraduate psychology degree courses in the UK.' *Psychology Teaching Review*, **5**(1996b): 40–6.

Further reading

Ferber, R. *Solve Your Child's Sleep Problems.* (London: Dorling Kindersley, 1986).

Quine, L. *Solving Children's Sleep Problems. A Step by Step Guide for Parents.* (Huntingdon: Beckett Karlson, 1997).

10

SERVICE RESPONSES TO THE 'DOUBLE DISABILITY' OF DOWN'S SYNDROME AND ALZHEIMER'S DISEASE

Richard Marler

The much increased life expectancy of people with Down's syndrome in recent years, as a result of better health care, means that many now survive to middle age and some to old age. It has been known for a long time, however, that there is an association between Down's syndrome and premature ageing, in particular a suscepti-bility to the development of early-onset Alzheimer's disease.

For the first time in the history of learning disability, there is now a sizeable group of older people with Down's syndrome, a sizeable minority of whom will experience symptoms of Alzheimer's disease. The implications for individuals, carers and services are profound.

A primary concern is that, as people with Down's syndrome live longer and a growing number are identified as developing Alzheimer's disease at a relatively early age, services will be ill equipped to respond to their needs. Bauer and Shea (1986) put the point succinctly:

> Identification of Alzheimer's disease in adults with Down's syndrome is of little significance unless the information is applied to enhance services for these individuals, their families and care-givers. (p. 148)

One problem is that learning disability services are often geared to promoting and supporting an increased level of independence. The declining health and increasing support needs of some people appear to run contrary to the main thrust of service aims and objectives.

Moreover, services for older people may have difficulty accommodating people's learning difficulties and therefore be unable to respond to this doubly affected group. Marler and Cunningham (1994), in their guide for carers, summarise the difficulties thus:

A problem one often meets when trying to get services for people with Down's syndrome is finding a service that feels it can cope with the two disabilities. Services specialised in learning disability often feel they are not equipped to cope with the Alzheimer's disease and, conversely, those specialised in dementia and ageing feel ill-equipped to deal with the learning disability. Some of this is merely a problem of labels since many of the basic needs and methods of help are similar. (p. 23)

The inflexibility of current service models causes many people with Down's syndrome and Alzheimer's disease to fall between two stools.

However, before we look a little more closely at how services might respond more appropriately, we shall examine what is known about the Down's syndrome–Alzheimer's disease connection, making particular reference to diagnosis and care approaches. We shall then consider the author's small-scale study on the service needs of this group as seen by families and care professionals. Finally, we shall look at how services might make the necessary adjustments to meet the needs of this group of people affected by a 'double disability'.

The Down's syndrome–Alzheimer's disease connection

Life expectancy

The first dimension in the picture is the change in life expectancy of people with Down's syndrome. It is well known that people with Down's syndrome have an increased vulnerability to various illnesses, including heart disease, respiratory infections and immunodeficiency. In recent years, however, the advent of antibiotics, open heart surgery, immunisation programmes and better standards of general health care and treatment have had a major impact on the life expectancy of people with Down's syndrome.

Whereas the average life expectancy of people with Down's syndrome in 1929 was only 9 years, by the late 1980s it was projected that 70 per cent would survive to their thirties, with 44 per cent reaching 60 years of age and 13 per cent living to their late sixties (Baird and Sadovnik, 1988). As people with Down's syndrome live longer, however, many experience early ageing and a proportion succumb to Alzheimer's disease in mid-life (Berg *et al.*, 1993).

Genetic link

The connection between Down's syndrome and Alzheimer's disease has attracted great research interest, not least because it has seemed to offer a clue to an understanding of the nature of Alzheimer's disease itself. Research has concluded that the neuropathology of Alzheimer's disease is present in every person with Down's syndrome over the age of about 40 years, many developing the typical senile plaques and neurofibrillary tangles in the brain from their twenties. These plaques and tangles are made up of dead and dying brain tissue, and it is these which cause the memory loss, confusion and behavioural change that are characteristic of this form of dementia. Despite the universal presence of the brain pathology of Alzheimer's disease, it is not known why only a proportion of middle-aged and older people with Down's syndrome exhibit symptoms of the illness.

Research in recent years has also established that there is a genetic link between one type of Alzheimer's disease and chromosome 21. Since people with Down's syndrome have an extra chromosome 21, this may explain their particular vulnerability to developing the illness. It appears that a tiny genetic defect on chromosome 21 causes the build up of amyloid deposits in the brain. These deposits in turn create the accumulation of dead and dying cells in the form of plaques and tangles, which cause the characteristic loss of abilities of the person affected. Moreover, research has uncovered a familial connection between Alzheimer's disease and Down's syndrome, supporting the genetic link theory (Schupf *et al.*, 1994).

Despite some excitement in research circles that genetic manipulation will one day become possible and ways will be found to prevent the destruction of brain cells, there is as yet no known cure for Alzheimer's disease. Nevertheless, the research carried out on people with Down's syndrome has contributed greatly to the understanding of Alzheimer's disease and its aetiology. Inasmuch as people with Down's syndrome have helped research, it is hoped that one day they will in return be helped by research, when a treatment is finally discovered.

Incidence

Exactly what proportion of people with Down's syndrome develop Alzheimer's disease symptoms is a very unclear part of the picture. There are, surprisingly perhaps, no national statistics, and the findings from research studies have been extraordinarily disparate. This may reflect the difficulties in making a diagnosis, which will be referred to later. Studies in recent decades have, however, suggested that as many as 45 per cent of those aged 45 or over may be affected by Alzheimer's disease (Thase et al., 1982).

A study of all people with Down's syndrome living in Leicestershire found that the average age of onset of Alzheimer's disease was 54 years (Collacott et al., 1992). It seems that although mainly over 50-year-olds are affected, some younger individuals do develop symptoms. Even the most pessimistic findings, however, indicate that less than half the middle-aged Down's syndrome population will have the illness. Indeed, the author knows personally a number of people with Down's syndrome in their sixties and seventies who show no symptoms whatsoever and are leading full and active lives. Marler and Cunningham (1994) suggest that:

It may turn out that the same percentage of people with Down's syndrome become affected by Alzheimer's disease as in the general population – but from a much earlier age. (p. 11)

In conclusion, then, despite the universal presence of Alzheimer's disease neuropathology, only a proportion of people with Down's syndrome develop the condition. However, because people with Down's syndrome generally are living longer, a sizeable number are developing symptoms of the illness, typically from middle age onwards.

Diagnosis

A confirmed diagnosis of Alzheimer's disease can only be made on post mortem examination of brain tissue. Although the symptoms of Alzheimer's disease may seem dramatic, the early signs may be masked by the person's learning difficulties and other impairments such as deterioration in vision or hearing. Indeed, sensory deficits are known to be far more common in older people with Down's syndrome and may contribute to a decline in abilities (Roeden and Zitman, 1995).

Despite the development of new assessment tools, a lack of reliable tests for Alzheimer's disease in people with learning difficulties may explain the disparate findings of research studies into its incidence. Moreover, other conditions that can cause similar symptoms, such as hypothyroidism and depression, have been highlighted as being associated with Down's syndrome (DoH, 1995; Prasher, 1995). Since these conditions are treatable, it is vitally important that carers seek a full medical assessment at an early stage.

After disorders such as hypothyroidism and depression have been excluded by the medical profession, changes in the individual's abilities and behaviour will be considered to see whether they are consistent with symptoms of Alzheimer's disease. A brain scan is sometimes suggested to see whether there has been cortical atrophy, although this will be only one factor in arriving at a tentative decision. The involvement of a consultant in learning disability and/or psychogeriatrics is likely to be suggested by a person's general practitioner when considering a diagnosis.

Studies on Down's syndrome and Alzheimer's disease indicate that, despite individual differences, people with Down's syndrome who have this sort of dementia show similar symptoms and stages to those of other people with Alzheimer's disease, although they may appear somewhat different because of their learning difficulties and different lifestyles. Common symptoms include:

- global impairments of daily living and self-care skills;
- disorientation, memory loss and restlessness;
- a lost ability to recognise the significance of what is seen, heard or felt;
- a loss of cognitive function;
- a loss of communication and spontaneity;
- fatigue, apathy and slowing down;
- increased stubbornness, mood change and depression;
- loss of mobility, and sleep disturbance;
- epilepsy, weight loss and incontinence.

Although Dalton and Wisniewski (1990), in their review, maintain that the literature is silent on psychiatric symptoms, Oliver and Holland (1986) found that difficult behaviour and mood lability were recorded in some studies. A more recent study by Prasher and Filer (1995) found that behavioural disturbance was common among people with Down's syndrome and Alzheimer's disease, but, interestingly, aggressive behaviour was infrequent. Nevertheless, most studies conclude that people with Down's syndrome and Alzheimer's disease show symptoms and stages similar to those of other people with Alzheimer's disease, although death from other age-related causes may occur before the full clinical signs of dementia appear.

There may be very gradual changes over a long period that are not recognised until after a particular event. In the author's experience, such events have been known to include:

- a near accident caused by the loss of ability to cross roads;
- a loss of former domestic skills, for example making tea without a tea bag;
- repetitive actions such as frequent changing of bed linen or putting on several sets of clothing.

Short-term alterations in someone's behaviour may be related to all kinds of change in someone's living situation, but deterioration over a period of time is important to note as this may be more likely to relate to the Alzheimer's condition. Even when a diagnosis of Alzheimer's disease is made, it is important to recognise that treatment may help with some symptoms. For example, the onset of epilepsy, which seems to be a common feature in people with Down's syndrome and Alzheimer's disease, may require treatment with anticonvulsants. There is also a danger of all the symptoms being attributed to Alzheimer's disease without treatment being sought. The author knows of a situation, for example, in which hearing impairment was put down to Alzheimer's disease before discovering that the cause was excessive ear wax!

Although everyone with Alzheimer's disease shares common symptoms and stages, each person follows their own individual path through the illness, this also being true for people with Down's syndrome. They will progressively lose their skills and abilities, some at a fast pace, others at a slow one, while yet others will experience 'plateaux' – periods when their symptoms remain stable.

Care approaches

There is an increasing literature on approaches to people with Down's syndrome who develop Alzheimer's symptoms (Marler and Cunningham, 1994), and much can be learned from the approaches recommended for those affected in the general population (Lay and Woods, 1996).

Various suggestions have been made to help people to maintain their existing skills, such as simplification of routines and memory aids – for example, the use of a calendar to record daily events and establishing one place to keep keys and important items. Help should be geared towards allowing clients to do as much as possible for themselves, assisting them only where necessary and not 'taking over' tasks. Making decisions easier by, for example, leaving out clothes can make self-care tasks more manageable. Seemingly over-whelming problems, for example the prevention of napping and increased exercise to overcome poor sleeping patterns, can be tackled.

Reminiscence – exploiting the familiarity of the past by visiting old friends and places, talking over past achievements and looking at old photos – is useful to people in whom an ageing process is taking place and may be very appropriate with older people with Down's syndrome. Helping people to make a photographic record of their own history has been suggested as a helpful activity.

Reality orientation programmes and environments stimulating people to relearn the basic facts about themselves and the world around them have also been recommended (Prosser, 1989). Some sensitivity is required, however, to avoid creating additional confusion and distress. Carers also need to adjust their communication patterns with people who may be losing their skills, and it has been suggested that more eye-to-eye contact, a slowing of communication and an increased use of touching may be helpful (Bauer and Shea, 1986).

Services – traditional patterns

As suggested earlier, the needs of people with Down's syndrome and Alzheimer's disease do not necessarily fit the services available. This is because many people with Down's syndrome develop the illness at an earlier age than do the general population.

Normalisation theory may suggest that middle-aged people with Down's syndrome and Alzheimer's disease should receive the same services as other people with early-onset dementia. The reality is, however, that in many areas, such services are based on the needs of the (larger) group of elderly people affected by the illness. Services for mainly elderly people may, on the one hand, appear unsuitable for a younger person, and on the other, actually be denied to someone with Down's syndrome because of his or her learning difficulties.

Another socially valued option, that of staying in one's accustomed place of residence with additional support services being provided, may also be denied to an individual affected by this 'double disability'. This may be because, as suggested earlier, learning disability services tend to be geared to supporting greater levels of functioning. The needs of a person with deteriorating health and abilities may sit uncomfortably within service philosophies. As Marshall (1992) points out:

> They risk being passed like hot potatoes between and within services, with no service really able to meet their needs. (p. 25)

Some people with Down's syndrome will be living with their families, who will have the uncomfortable dilemma of whether to attempt to cope at home or to seek residential care. Although the NHS and Community Care Act 1990 has shifted the balance of care from residential to supported care in people's own homes, whether important support services such as day care, respite care and home care are made available nevertheless depends very much on local social services budgets. People with Down's syndrome and Alzheimer's disease therefore do not seem to fit neatly into how services are organised and many fall between them.

Author's study

In an attempt to look at the service issues for people with Down's syndrome who develop Alzheimer's disease, the author conducted a small-scale research study (Marler, 1992). This examined the experience of 20 affected people living in the south of England. It involved interviewing the care givers, family members and key professionals concerned with each individual. Because of the nature of the illness, it was not possible to obtain the views of the people with Down's syndrome directly. The areas covered by interview included:

- the history of the illness, changes in health, abilities and behaviour, and details of the diagnosis;
- a knowledge of the connection between Down's syndrome and Alzheimer's disease;

- service provision, appropriateness and requirements;
- the experience of giving care and obtaining services;
- suggestions for service improvements.

Although this study involved a small sample, needs ranged from low dependency for people at the early stages of Alzheimer's disease to high dependency for people in the later stages of the illness. In the course of the study, three individuals in the sample died, which was a stark reminder of the nature of the study.

People in the sample were living in a range of situations – family homes, residential homes for people with learning difficulties, and nursing/rest homes for elderly people. Although those living in nursing homes were heavily dependent, other equally dependent people were living in social services or voluntary sector homes, or at home with family members.

Case studies

Before describing the results of this study, three case studies are summarised below in order to illustrate the types of situation faced by people in the sample. Names have been changed out of respect for privacy.

CASE STUDY 1
NANCY

This 61-year-old woman with Down's syndrome lives with her older sister, Theresa, who made a promise to her mother before her death not to let Nancy go into residential care. Nancy was always an easy person to live with, sociable, friendly and helpful around the house, but about two and a half years ago, another sister who lives nearby noticed that Nancy was becoming noticeably quieter, less lively and with less sparkle to her personality. Both sisters put it down to Nancy 'getting older'. Then, 2 years ago and out of the blue, she had an epileptic fit. Tests followed, and it was then that the diagnosis of Alzheimer's disease was made. It came as a big shock to the sisters, who were vaguely aware that people with Down's syndrome have a shorter life expectancy but were ignorant of the connection with Alzheimer's disease.

Since then, although good days follow bad, the general picture is one of decline. Her sisters refer to the 'AD curtain' coming down, and then Nancy cries a lot, becomes frustrated and pushes people away when she does not want to do something. She wanders aimlessly from place to place, talking to the carpet or imaginary people in the garden. She has lost some of her washing, dressing and eating skills, and has become less mobile. Theresa, who has arthritis, is often exhausted by the physical and emotional demands of caring for her sister.

A specialist social worker visits and negotiates for services. She has found that it is very much a case of testing out, of seeing who can provide the best service, because Nancy does not fit neatly into the services provided. Respite care at a home for people with learning difficulties failed because of an inadequate staff level. A day centre for people with Alzheimer's disease needed to be persuaded to give Nancy a trial, but she now attends one day a week and is popularly seen as the 'life and soul' of the place. The staff there maintain that she has needs very different from those of the other clients, although the social worker wonders whether this is just because she looks different. Respite care is available on the same site.

Nancy's sisters are not at all convinced that she should be with very elderly people and are not happy with the respite care facilities. Social services home care and a Good Neighbours scheme help with dressing, bathing and washing Nancy's hair three times a week, although help is really needed on a daily basis. Theresa would like a sitter service so that she can go shopping without having to rely on Nancy being co-operative.

It seems to Theresa that voluntary groups concentrate on youngsters moving on to greater independence and opportunities, and she feels there is not the same interest in older people with learning difficulties. Despite the help from her family and local services, Nancy and her sister feel very isolated.

CASE STUDY 2
CHARLES

Charles is a 42-year-old man with Down's syndrome who, until recently, was living in a social services home several miles away from where his parents live. He had a relatively independent lifestyle, going out to pubs, swimming pools and football grounds on his own and indulging in his love for photography. He developed alopecia at an early age but has coped well with taunts of 'baldy' from local children.

About three and a half years ago, some concern was expressed about his tiredness and the fact that he would sometimes fall asleep at the workshop he attended. Staff in the home, however, were so confident in his abilities that he was moved to a training flat within the home to prepare for independence in the community. He had his own furniture there and was for a time very happy. Then he began to come home to his parents with strange stories about people trying to get him into their cars in the middle of the night. He started wandering off from the workshop, giving further cause for concern.

The news of the opening of a new Mencap home near his parents' house seemed to offer the answer to the problem of his parents keeping a closer eye on him – and Charles wanted to apply. He started to attend a different day centre, near the new home, where he was happy, but he became confused about the journey from the old home. His parents decided that it would be best if he came to live with them until the new home was ready.

Charles, however, became more and more withdrawn and irrational. One of his chores was laying the table, which he could always do perfectly for any number of people and for any meal. He started to get up in the middle of the night to do this.

He eventually moved into the home but, on the first weekend, attacked another resident and wrecked the lounge. Prior to this, the most violent thing he had ever done was to slam a door. He was treated for depression without success, and finally, after a brain scan, Alzheimer's disease was diagnosed by the local consultant in learning disability. Attempts to reintroduce Charles to the home failed as his mental condition deteriorated quickly.

Charles' parents struggled on for a further 6 months. Sometimes he refused to get up in the mornings, and he was needing more and more help with toileting and bathing. The offer of a place in a large NHS Trust learning disability residential unit was received with alarm by his parents, who knew that it was too large and noisy for their son. A community nurse from the local community team for people with learning difficulties (CTPLD) introduced them to a nursing home specialising in care for people with Alzheimer's disease and which had experience of people with Down's syndrome. Reluctantly, Charles' parents agreed for him to move, and they have continued to visit him there daily.

Since then, Charles has had a number of epileptic fits, becoming less and less communicative and more and more dependent. For periods, he refuses to eat or drink. The CTPLD's speech and language therapist and a psychologist in elderly services have become involved in order to give advice to the nursing home staff. The community nurse attempted reminiscence work with Charles by bringing in photos, but he turned his head and seemed to want to cut himself off from his past.

Although they are appreciative of the care Charles receives, his parents are distressed to see their 42-year-old son living with very elderly demented people and progressively losing his abilities.

CASE STUDY 3
FRANK

At the age of 40, Frank moved into a residential community run by a voluntary organisation, having been the sole carer of his elderly mother until shortly before her death.

He surprised those who had fixed images of people with Down's syndrome, by being very articulate and very capable. He travelled daily by public transport between the community home and a craft workshop, where he designed and made rugs to a highly skilled level. He impressed people with his wit and sense of humour, his spiritual faith and his capacity to accept life as it came.

At the age of 49, however, Frank began to forget people's names and became generally more absent minded. This was followed by a period of slowing down and some unusual incidents, such as changing the sheets on his bed three times on a Saturday instead of once. He had some insight into his problems and asked his carers to tell him what was wrong with him.

Three years later, Frank suffered a major fit for the first time in his life, simultaneously with what appeared to be a stroke. After that, there was a massive deterioration, Frank becoming less mobile and less communicative, as well as losing his writing ability and some of his self-care skills. He went on to have fits and minor strokes, losing a bit more ability each time. Frank continued to attend the workshop, but increasingly for social reasons, as designing rug patterns dwindled to doodling and eventually scribbling on his clothes.

Then Frank began to have hallucinations and see flamingos on the ceiling of his bedroom. He no longer recognised the house as his home, and at times thought his mum was alive or, more distressingly, had just died. 'I'd like to go home now please', he would say. He went on to become less polite and, out of character, somewhat aggressive. Although there were enormous difficulties, the voluntary organisation was committed to continuing to care for him in the home that had been his for 14 years.

Because climbing stairs became difficult, Frank's bedroom was moved downstairs, although this disorientated him. He became restless at night-time and needed considerably more personal care.

Help was sought from a range of professionals. When the diagnosis of Alzheimer's disease had been made, a consultant in learning disability gave the staff team some useful preparation in terms of information, advice and support. At a later stage, when it was evident that Frank was deteriorating quickly, a psychiatrist attempted to support them both by looking at issues of bereavement and loss. Frank's GP was caring and mobilised other services. A district nurse came once a week to bath and check Frank, but more importantly invited the assistants to unburden themselves to her about the difficulties of looking after someone with Alzheimer's disease.

A major source of help came from the local community learning disability team, which provided physiotherapy, occupational therapy and community nursing support. One failure in service provision was the adaptation of the house's bathroom to Frank's needs. Although the need had been identified for a year, the bureaucracy involved in getting technical advice and financial assistance was inordinately time-consuming, and the adaptations were in fact never carried out. Another problem was night-time care, which was difficult to cater for with fixed staffing levels and no domiciliary night nursing service in the area.

It became clear that Frank's deterioration was relentless. Although the physical demands of caring for Frank were stressful, it was the fear of facing his death that created the most tension for staff and residents alike. When it came, however, Frank's death seemed very natural.

On his last night, when it was clear that he was dying, those who indicated a wish to, took it in turn to sit with him, saying goodbye in their own way. Frank's death was not terrifying but was seen as the most natural thing in the world. Those who wanted to, came and saw his body and said their last goodbyes. One resident prayed that Frank would still get his Christmas presents in heaven. Others brought flowers and touched him. The whole community came together in prayers, sharing tales about Frank and celebrating his life.

Results of the author's study

Knowledge of the connection

The people involved in caring for individuals with Down's syndrome and Alzheimer's disease – like Nancy, Charles and Frank – were asked whether they knew about the connection between Down's syndrome and Alzheimer's disease before their individual was diagnosed. While 75 per cent of the outside professionals interviewed, and about 33 per cent of direct care staff, had previously known about the connection, all those who had not known felt that they needed to know.

Among family members, in contrast, there was a complete absence of previous knowledge about the connection. As in Nancy's case, the diagnosis of Alzheimer's disease for their relatives had come as a complete surprise and shock. Unlike care staff and other professionals, however, they were not unanimous in feeling that they should have known before the event. The reason for this varied from 'There's no cure, so why know in advance?' to 'I've always looked for the positives in having a daughter with Down's syndrome; I wouldn't have wanted to face such a negative before I had to.'

This poses a certain dilemma for professional staff working with families in which there is a member with Down's syndrome. Sensitivity is clearly needed in deciding whether or not to inform families.

All those interviewed did, however, feel that they lacked knowledge about the condition after the diagnosis of Alzheimer's disease had been made. They wanted further information in order better to carry out the caring task. Marler and Cunningham (1994) responded to this by collaborating with the Down's Syndrome Association to produce a guide for carers.

Residential services

The people in this sample lived in a range of residential settings. In the course of interviewing, it emerged that over half of the people with higher-dependency needs had had to move as a direct result of developing Alzheimer's disease symptoms; the placements of some individuals in the early stages were also threatened. Frank's situation – in which his carers were committed to caring for him throughout the illness – was exceptional.

Reservations were expressed about the suitability of nursing or rest home provision for people with Down's syndrome under pensionable age (as in Charles' case). These reservations, focusing on the lack of individual attention and the very elderly population in these homes, came from families, professionals and nursing home staff themselves. Most carers felt that, ideally, the individual affected should 'stay put', additional resources being provided. If, however, they really did have to move, it should be to small, quiet residential homes with other older people with learning difficulties. In general, carers expressed little preference for whether the statutory or independent sector should provide this type of facility.

Day care services

Day care, or a lack of it, was seen as a major issue by those interviewed. Almost half of the sample had no day care at all, and several more received only a part-time service. Most day care was provided in social education centres or special care units with other people with learning difficulties. Only one person (Nancy) attended a day centre for elderly confused people, several others having been refused similar services because of their visible learning difficulties.

Most respondents felt that their individuals needed to receive day care support in small groups in quiet environments with therapeutic approaches based on reminiscence and reality orientation. Some felt that learning disability services needed to provide such groups; others felt that services for elderly people or mixed client groups might be equally appropriate.

Support services

Care givers were asked what professional support services were provided at the time and what additional professional services were, in their opinion, required. In general, it became clear that respondents felt that the problems engendered by the needs of someone with Down's syndrome and Alzheimer's disease required help from a range of professionals rather than just one. Families looked to specialists in learning disability services to provide support, and CTPLDs were generally complimented for offering a coordinated range of professional input. The potential contribution of professionals specialising in work with elderly people, and with expertise in the management of Alzheimer's disease, was recognised by professionals in learning disability services.

Problems in obtaining respite care were identified by several family carers, and this had contributed to the decision to seek residential care for some individuals. The problem related to finding services that met both sets of needs – those arising from learning difficulties and those caused by Alzheimer's disease.

Home care services were reported to be more flexible and supportive than carers had expected, although the need was pinpointed for more 'sitter-type' services to allow the carer to leave the home occasionally (as Nancy's sister wanted).

Some carers had experienced a considerable delay in obtaining necessary adaptations and equipment.

Services – new patterns

Because of individual differences and because of the individual pattern of the illness, a range of services needs to be offered to people with Down's syndrome who develop Alzheimer's disease. Any model of service provision, therefore, needs to include alternative options and choices.

What is clear, however, is that learning disability services need to adjust their remit to include the needs of people who are losing skills rather than focusing only on the training of people for greater and greater independence. Supporting people with deteriorating health and abilities seems to go against the grain of current services. There thus needs to be a sea change in how learning disability services are provided.

The author's study suggested that people with Down's syndrome who develop Alzheimer's symptoms should, ideally, 'stay put', especially in view of the fact that change can exacerbate the condition. Despite the enormous difficulties for carers and fellow residents, the study found examples of residential homes that had been able to secure additional support and make the necessary adjustments. For those living in the family home, much-increased home care services, together with adequate day and respite services, are needed to support family members in the caring task. For those living in residential care, every effort should be made for extra resources to be redirected to the individual's current living situation rather than their having to move. The provision of additional resources to allow someone to remain in a familiar environment is indeed consistent with community care policy.

Should a move become desirable, however, it has been suggested that while nursing homes may be suitable for older people, they may not be ideal for middle-aged people with Down's syndrome. Small, quiet residential homes with other older people with learning difficulties have been suggested as a better alternative. Such provision needs to be developed by the statutory or independent sector. More importantly, a change of attitude is needed in both learning disability services and those for elderly people so that there can be some flexibility of provision to respond to individual needs.

CTPLDs clearly need to inform themselves about the needs of this doubly affected group as they have a crucial role in coordinating professional support to care givers. Links with services to people in the general population who develop Alzheimer's disease also need to be made.

The requirement laid down by the NHS and Community Care Act 1990 that social services departments formulate local community care plans, in collaboration with health authorities and NHS Trusts, the independent sector and user groups, is an opportunity for proper plans to be made. Joint commissioning or unified systems of services delivery will also benefit this group of people whose needs straddle traditional service boundaries.

If this opportunity is not taken, an increasing number of people with Down's syndrome who develop Alzheimer's disease will not receive the services they merit or the care they deserve.

Checklist for action

- Care givers need to be made aware of the symptoms of Alzheimer's disease and its connection with Down's syndrome.
- Careful note should be made of significant changes in the health, behaviour and abilities of an individual with Down's syndrome over a period of time.
- A full medical assessment should be sought in the event of concern, and attention given to treatable symptoms.
- In the event of a diagnosis of Alzheimer's disease, care givers need to adjust their approach to supporting an individual's level of functioning.

- Services need to be adjusted to meet a different set of needs, allowing, wherever possible, the individual with Down's syndrome to 'stay put'.
- Both learning disability services and services for older people need to adjust their remits to include the needs of ageing people with learning difficulties and to provide additional services.
- Communication between the two services needs to be enhanced.
- Local community care plans should spell out how the needs of this doubly disabled group will be addressed.

References

Baird, P. and Sadovnik, A. 'Life expectancy in Down's syndrome adults.' *Lancet*, 10 December (1988): 1354–6.

Bauer, A. and Shea, T. 'Alzheimer's disease and Down's syndrome: a review and implications for adult services.' *Education and Training of the Mentally Retarded*, June (1986): 144–50.

Berg, J., Karlinsky, H. and Holland, A. *Alzheimer's Disease, Down's Syndrome and their Relationship*. (Oxford: Oxford Medical Publications, 1993).

Collacott, R., Cooper, S. and McGrother, C. 'Differential rates of psychiatric disorders in adults with Down's syndrome compared with other mentally handicapped adults.' *British Journal of Psychiatry*, 161(1992): 671–4.

Dalton, A. and Wisniewski, H. 'Down's syndrome and the dementia of Alzheimer's disease.' *International Review of Psychiatry*, 2(1990): 43–52.

Department of Health. *The Health of the Nation: A Strategy for People with Learning Disabilities.* (London: HMSO, 1995).

Lay, C. and Woods, R. *Caring for the Person with Dementia: A Guide for Families and Other Carers* (4th edn). (London: Alzheimer's Disease Society, 1996).

Marler, R. The service needs of people with Down's syndrome who develop Alzheimer's disease. Unpublished research thesis. (Portsmouth: University of Portsmouth, 1992).

Marler, R. and Cunningham, C. *Down's Syndrome and Alzheimer's Disease: A Guide for Carers*. (London: Down's Syndrome Association, 1994).

Marshall, M. 'Down's syndrome and dementia', in CCETSW *A Double Challenge: Working with People who have both Learning Difficulties and a Mental Illness.* CCETSW Paper No. 19.27. (London: Central Council for Education and Training in Social Work, 1992).

Oliver, C. and Holland, A. 'Down's syndrome and Alzheimer's disease: a review.' *Psychological Medicine*, 16(1986): 307–22.

Prasher, V. 'Differential diagnosis between Alzheimer's disease and hypothyroidism in adults with Down's syndrome.' *Down's Syndrome Research and Practice*, 3(i)(1995): 15–18.

Prasher, V. and Filer, A. 'Behavioural disturbance in people with Down's syndrome and dementia.' *Journal of Intellectual Research*, **39**(5)(1995): 432–6.

Prosser, G. 'Down's syndrome, Alzheimer's disease and reality orientation: a review.' *Mental Handicap*, **17**(1989): 50–3.

Roeden, J. and Zitman, F. 'Ageing in adults with Down's syndrome in institutionally based and community based residences.' *Journal of Intellectual Disability Research*, **39**(5)(1995): 399–407.

Schupf, N., Kampel, D., Lee, J., Ottman, R. and Mayeux, R. 'Increased risk of Alzheimer's disease in mothers of adults with Down's syndrome.' *Lancet*, **344**(1994): 353–6.

Thase, M., Liss, L., Smeltzer, D. and Maloon, J. 'Clinical evaluation of dementia in Down's syndrome: a preliminary report.' *Journal of Mental Deficiency Research*, **26**(1982): 239–44.

11

NUTRITION STANDARDS IN SMALL COMMUNITY HOUSES

Karen Jeffereys

Current health policies continue to acknowledge the importance of diet on the nation's health. Published and unpublished research shows that people with learning difficulties have a high risk of being nutritionally compromised. There remains, however, a gap between this knowledge, health policy and the appropriate action. This author advocates that addressing the nutrition standards in residential houses through organisational approaches could significantly and positively improve the quality of life for people with learning difficulties. An organisational approach is novel as it has not previously been discussed in the literature. This text describes the current situation as well as reviewing research and audit in the UK and abroad. The intent is to share a broad range of issues, highlighting possible applications and expanding the awareness among providers and purchasers of services.

Introduction

Social policy and hospital enquiries since the mid-1970s have enabled people with a learning difficulty to move from institutions to alternative accommodation in the community. Within the considerations of such major changes, and the impact that they would have upon people's lives, nutrition and catering (food services) received little attention.

Two assumptions were perhaps made. First was that the negative social and nutritional aspects of large-scale institutionalised catering would be replaced with positive ones of domestic 'family'-style catering. Second, community care policy would automatically meet people's nutritional needs. Alternatively, policy makers and service planners perhaps followed a historical path, giving little consideration to providing quality food services.

It is only recently that the Department of Health (DoH) has addressed nutrition standards in acute hospitals (NHS Executive, 1996) and that the Royal College of Nursing has developed nutrition standards for older adults, a group of people known to be nutritionally at risk (RCN, 1993). However, research into and the monitoring of people's nutritional status and the nutrition standards within community accommodation for people with learning difficulties has not been considered at a national level. Sadly, local NHS health Trusts have varied in their concern and commitment to this issue. The shift of overall responsibility, from people trained in catering and nutrition to people who have little or no formal training, has received inadequate attention. Few Trusts have adequately resourced their service with professionals to facilitate quality food services.

A survey carried out by the author in 1992 showed that 72 dietitians were employed by 65 Trusts to provide dietetic services for adults with learning difficulties (British Dietetic Association, 1993). Eighty-four per cent of these were part-time posts, averaging 0.38 whole-time equivalents, but 64 per cent shared this time between children and adults with learning difficulties. Work has not been carried out to define how many dietitians are needed per 1000 population of adults with learning difficulties. However, these figures strongly suggest an inadequate resourcing of dietitians in this area. Additionally, the closure of large hospitals has resulted in budget savings by employing fewer catering managers. A number of Trusts still do not employ skilled people to facilitate quality food services in community accommodation for people with learning difficulties.

Despite these figures, the author believes that the providers of small community housing care about nutrition. Planners' knowledge of the issues surrounding food services, however, limits their interpretation and the appropriate resourcing. The issues obviously differ depending upon the current and previous catering services. Variables include the presence of a trained cook, the house staff, the people who live in the house (householders) and Cook Chill food services. Although many of the issues described are pertinent to all food services and types of accommodation, they will not be alluded to in this text. The focus of this chapter is small community houses where support workers and householders are responsible for the day-to-day food services (self-catering). In addition, the focus of research and strategies for implementing nutrition standards is within health Trust community houses.

Definition

Clarifying the term 'nutrition standards' has not been attempted in the literature, and it has thus been widely interpreted. With no other description to relate to, the author asserts that comprehensive nutrition standards describe the aspects of a person's life that will influence his or her enjoyment of food, levels of independence, nutritional status and overall health and wellbeing. Services should address four key areas (Table 11.1) in order to provide nutritionally adequate diets and to observe householders' rights.

Table 11.1   Key areas of comprehensive nutrition standards

Area	Aspect
Independence and self-advocacy	Choice
	Participation
Environment	Hygiene
	Dining room
	Staff attitudes
	Community presence
Food quality	Hygiene
	Catering skills
	Nutritional content
Nutritional health	Nutrition screening
	Weight
	Medical problems, for example constipation
	Drug–nutrient interaction

Are standards necessary?

A service driven by normalisation philosophy may argue that people living in small houses should have the same access to food as other people. However, defining 'the same access to food as other people' is difficult when describing the nation's eating patterns. Additionally, justification for nutrition standards is required because, as a nation, we do not possess nutrition standards in our own homes. Conversely, a service driven by health philosophy may aim to meet people's nutritional needs but limit choice, participation and enjoyment. Food naturally falls into both the social care and health models; it cannot be separated and should include both service philosophies. It is therefore the responsibility of all providers, regardless of agency or social/health care model, to be able to monitor the nutrition standards of their houses. Irrespective of business direction, the opportunities and limitations in achieving such a task are the same.

Consumer rights are of prime consideration as it is not 'normal' to have nutrition standards in one's own home. However, in circumstances in which people live together and eat in a group, it would be usual for householders to have some form of mutually agreed 'rules', even if unwritten. Given the choice, people would base these on life experiences, knowledge, food beliefs, skills, finance, facilities and access to food. Potentially diverse experiences coexist in residential houses, those of householders and those of staff. Undoubtedly, staff may, although they mean well, inflict their food perceptions and habits upon others.

These issues were reported by Wallace (1995, p. 23) in her needs assessment report. She found that staff challenged the need to develop food service guidelines for people with mental illness in community houses – 'why should mental illness... single them out from the rest of the community? Another important point raised was the fact that staff's personal values impact upon the residents' own values'.

Although Wallace's work focused upon mental health services, it supports the notion that standards are necessary, in circumstances in which people's rights might be marginalised, in order to provide a consistent and acceptable food service. In fact, it may be more important for people with learning difficulties who may have limited food experiences, communication skills and control over their lives. Additionally, standards could prevent the abdication of responsibility that may occur when normalisation principles are quoted. It is true that all people have the right to eat whatever they want, when and where and with whom they want, but it is dereliction of duty not to help people to make informed choices, and not to make positive opportunities available.

The aim of developing nutrition standards is to ensure that a nutritionally adequate diet is offered. Nutrition standards should aim to meet individuals' needs, optimising their physical health, participation, choice and enjoyment. Stand-alone dogmatic statements on the quality or quantity of particular foods will have little impact unless they are woven into the context of people's lives.

National and international perspective

In 1991, the author personally reviewed the tools used to measure quality of care and/or life for people with learning difficulties; this elicited little evidence that nutrition had been considered. Some tools (National Development Group for Mentally Handicapped, 1980; Ager, 1986) contained a small number of items related to the nutrition and food service. Only the USA had a statutory tool (Department of Health and Human Services, 1988) with which to evaluate this area in any depth. Interestingly, a number of workers commented, in response to the author's communication, that nutrition-related issues had been unconsciously omitted, but they acknowledged their importance.

The Registered Homes Act

British legislation (Registered Homes Act 1984) states the requirements for registered homes. While the Act provides guidelines, it does not direct registered home owners or inspectors towards objective food service standards. Regulations 6(1), Schedule 2(8), Regulation 9(1) and Regulation 10(1k, 1l) all relate to food services. The latter regulation addresses the 'Provision of facilities and services', stating that:

> the person registered shall having regard to the size of the home and number, age, sex and condition of residents... (l) supply suitable, varied and properly prepared wholesome and nutritious food in adequate quantities for residents.

The intent behind these regulations is certainly for registered home owners to provide high-quality services, but it depends entirely upon local interpretation. Inspectorate teams may employ a different emphasis in their interpretation. For example, what are suitable, varied, properly prepared, wholesome, nutritious and adequate? The Centre for Policy on Ageing (1996) documents what is perceived as best practice and guides residential and nursing homes inspectors. Its book focuses upon older people in residential accommodation, but a similar publication addressing specific issues for people with learning difficulties does not exist. Unlike its predecessor (Centre for Policy on Ageing, 1984), it has not yet won ministerial acknowledgement. It is believed that the Department of Social

Services awaits the publication of the Registered Forum Standards by the Social Care Association, which will possibly relate to a wider range of people's needs.

Although community health houses are not registered, the Registered Homes Act 1984 provides a useful inception for those wishing to develop nutrition standards.

The King's Fund

The King's Fund (1996) has responded by developing organisational standards and criteria as well as a monitoring process for community services. The manual provides a baseline self-assessment tool to be used by organisations in order to audit their service against standards and criteria deemed to be best practice. Volume 1 focuses upon user rights and individual needs, while Volume 2 contains core and specific standards.

Catering services are among the 'Support Services Specific Standards' (p. 137–9). Standard 1 states 'The catering service provides a high quality service to patients/clients/users, staff and visitors in accordance with the people served' (p. 137). The criteria focus mainly upon the management of catering services and food safety, although one refers to nutrition: 'Menus are planned in discussion with the dietetic service, to provide meals which meet the needs of the patients and staff on either restricted or therapeutic diets' (p. 138). The guidance attached to this criteria draws attention to presentation, portion size, variety, cultural preference, special patient populations and menu cycles.

Although specific regard is paid to food provision, the criteria highlight issues for a catering service rather than self-catering houses. Additionally, they focus on special dietary needs rather than the nutritional needs of individual people. National dietary targets are not reflected in any of the criteria. However, health promotion is highlighted in Volume 2 in the 'Human Resources' section: 'Policies are developed which encourage the general health of patients/clients/users and staff. These include... Health of the Nation targets (where applicable)' (6.43, p. 40).

It is obvious that a useful audit tool cannot encompasses every area in depth without becoming repetitive and loathsome. However, a statement such as 'Nutrition standards, specific to the needs of the patient/client/user will be developed' might meet the needs of more people than might concentrating on specialist diets. The guidance brief could highlight nutritional adequacy, national dietary targets, user and staff involvement, choice, participation and facilities. This tool, recommendable as it is, certainly requires attention to issues surrounding food services in small community houses.

Dietitians' response

Some UK dietitians have appraised their local situation and, in the absence of concise national regulations, responded in different ways. Progress has been hampered by the lack of dietitians and by contracts specifying clinical rather than staff training and health promotion activities. Those who have begun developing standards have been driven by professional self-motivation rather than a learning disability service planner/purchaser directive. As a consequence, work in the UK has been developed in isolation. In some cases, the standards written have described the type and quantity of food/drink; others describe professional dietetic standards. Few address issues of choice, participation and enjoyment. A professional resource pack is being compiled in order to facilitate the sharing of work between dietitians (British Dietetic Association, 2000).

International interpretation

The author's correspondence with Australia, Canada and New Zealand provides useful insights for UK services. Unfortunately, little is published in the literature.

Canada

Soneff et al. (1994) describe their work to improve the quality of the food service in small facilities for adult care in British Colombia, Canada. They report that nutrition and food service regulations (Ministry of Health, 1991) must be met by all licensed facilities in order to operate:

Adherence to regulations and maintenance of standards provide a level of confidence that residents receive adequate nutrition care. They require, however, that facilities develop and follow policies and procedures regarding aspects of food service management. (Soneff et al. 1994, p. 869)

Interestingly, although ministry resources are available, Soneff suggests that they present several disadvantages to staff, for example expense, access, comprehension and inappropriate content. Their pilot survey strongly suggested a low compliance with these regulations.

As a result, Soneff *et al.* developed an audit tool to measure the effectiveness of two training methods. They compared three groups: those receiving the *Food Services Management Manual*, houses receiving the manual plus training and a control group receiving neither. The manual was modified from the province's policy documents on quality assurance, standards and regulations (Ministry of Health, 1991). They found no effect upon food purchasing and food storage. However, a significant improvement in audit scores for menu planning and food safety occurred in those receiving training workshops plus the manual compared with those who received the manual alone. No house scored the Gold Standard, set at 75 per cent.

They concluded that:

the usefulness of a manual alone is questionable... a workshop plus manual is the absolute minimum training strategy, and long-term follow up is essential... a well planned food service training program is ongoing, comprehensive, and must meet the performance expectations of the job. (p. 873)

They have now produced an extremely comprehensive *Food Service Manual for Small Facilities* (Soneff, 1991).

Australasia

In Australia, a human rights investigation into the treatment of the mentally ill criticised the state and federal governments for the number of services provided. Special funding purchased the Boarding House Project, which included the employment of a nutritionist and a 2-year project aimed 'to improve the nutritional status of SAHS residents with psychiatric disorders living in community residences' (Wallace, 1995, p. 2). Although the group of people considered in this project have mental illness, it again highlights potential problems when inadequate nutrition standards/legislation exist.

New Zealand dietitians are developing food and nutrition specifications for group homes, being in the process of submitting a draft to their purchaser of health with the aim of increasing the detail in the current specifications. The draft specification suggests that:

Every group home will have a written food and nutrition policy that covers the following issues: menu planning, nutrition and dietetic input, food safety, client involvement, inservice staff education relating to food and nutrition.

In addition, a dietitian working in the Public Health Service in the South Island is completing a manual for the care givers of people with intellectual disability and mental illness who live in group homes. The manual, *Living in the Community*, includes five sections: nutrition, meal planning, food safety, food skills and food choices. Soneff et al. (1994) have, however, clearly demonstrated the ineffectiveness of manuals alone.

Research

Published research describing the dietary intake and nutritional status of people with learning difficulties, although limited (Cunningham et al., 1990; Stewart et al., 1994; Caudrey and Russell, 1995), is greater in volume than that addressing the topic of nutrition standards. Three pieces of work specific to people with learning difficulties are known to the author. Two were undertaken by the author in Portsmouth between 1990 and 1993; the other is Soneff et al.'s work as described previously (1994).

Implementation: imposition or negotiation?

The first study (Hay and Jeffereys, 1992) focused upon methods of implementing nutrition standards in local community health houses. Two methods of introducing standards are to impose them upon and to negotiate with staff. It was the belief of the authors that managers, therapists and specialists normally impose policies, standards and/or recommendations on care staff and service users. This regrettably prevents the involvement of those providing or receiving the service. The other approach – negotiation – values experience and is more likely to produce practical, realistic standards. Hay and Jeffereys' (1992) small 2-year study explored the response of staff to dietitians imposing and negotiating nutrition standards.

Draft nutrition standards were developed by dietitians and introduced to two houses. The staff (and one householder) then modified them with the help of the dietitians. The final version contained four statements, each being subdivided into specific actions and monitoring procedures:

- Mealtimes and the availability of snacks and drinks should be as flexible as those found in a home situation.
- Staff should aim to provide a planned nutritionally adequate and varied diet suited to individual choice and requirements.
- The eating atmosphere should allow a relaxed, enjoyable social experience.
- Standards should undergo continual development, and a system of nutritional review for both home and individuals should be established to prevent stagnation and ensure maximum consistency.

The final standards were then imposed upon a similar pair of houses with no input from the dietitians. Both pairs of houses were directed that the standards should be monitored according to the monitoring instructions and evaluated in 2 months by the residential managers. A forum was held 1 month after the evaluation to conclude the study. This small forum presented the results of the study to all those involved, received their responses and asked 'Where do we go now?' The staff summarised four recommendations:

1. Nutrition standards should aim to establish a minimum requirement.
2. Nutrition standards must be negotiated with service users, staff and a dietitian. They should be individualised to each house.
3. Monitoring should be designed so that staff perform most of the tasks. The standard should be self-monitored, with dietetic liaison.
4. The implementation of nutrition standards can only be considered if a quality monitoring system exists and is used by the house.

Nutrition standards in seven houses

A second study (Jeffereys, 1993) provided a useful snapshot of nutrition standards in seven community health houses. Quantitative and qualitative data were collated, utilising two staff question-naires and observation methodology. The first questionnaire looked at general issues surrounding nutrition and quality of life issues, the second recording individual people's nutritional needs as perceived by their keyworker. The model, based upon Whittacker *et al.*'s (1991) work, used the experience of service users (research assistants) to carry out 2-day observations in each house.

Training

The training of the two research assistants was carried out infor-mally in social eating environments, cafés, home and pubs. Formal observation skills were further developed by 'dummy runs' in resi-dential accommodation of their own choice. Both chose hostels that they knew well and felt at ease in. One person chose her own home and was subsequently placed in a vulnerable position when criti-cism was fed back to staff. The repercussions for service users must certainly be considered when service users are involved in criticising their own services.

Results

The main nutrition findings showed that no forward menu planning occurred and that the principles by which meals were chosen varied between houses. Records of meals eaten were poor or non-existent in some houses. The frequency of meals and snacks was good, but fruit and vegetables were a limiting factor in the balance of meals offered. The intake of nutrients, such as vitamin D, calcium, iron and fibre, was low in some houses. Staff were aware of current low-fat, low-sugar, high-fibre principles but did not achieve the high-fibre principle in practice. Most people appeared to consume adequate fluids, but staff were less aware of the needs of those people who had increased requirements resulting from fluid loss.

Weights were recorded, but the method was inconsistent and not necessarily present in a comprehensive format. People's indi-vidual dietary requirements were generally understood and implemented for people who were identified as being overweight. However, documentation and practice for people who were underweight or had difficulty with certain food textures were inconsistent in some houses.

Staff placed value on choice and participation. Those people most able to express a choice were actively engaged in all aspects of meal choice and related food activities. People with profound learning difficulties were, however, less involved. The opportunity to make choices and participate in independent activities was most apparent at breakfast. Flexibility in terms of the place and timing of meals was evident in all houses. Most people in all the houses had the opportunity to eat a range of cuisine through the consumption of take aways or by eating out in community venues.

The dining room and kitchen environments were positively assessed by the research assistants, with the exception of two houses where the conditions were described as cramped.

The choice of method – to utilise the experience and skills of service users as observers – was positively received by the staff. Their total cooperation with the study and positive reception to the feedback of results strongly supports their desire to provide high-quality food services to the people who live in the houses. In addition, the sheer hard work and determination of the research assistants cannot be overestimated.

Portsmouth strategy

Lessons learnt from this local research placed Portsmouth Healthcare NHS Trust in a prime position to take action. Staff in these houses demonstrated a positive commitment, and their knowledge and skills were clearly an essential ingredient in the process of writing and achieving standards. However, in order to utilise staff skills, training and assessment tools were necessary. Subsequently, three major initiatives were undertaken: a training programme, nutrition screening and a Trust-wide Feeding People policy.

Catering skills course

This course was initiated by the catering advisor and dietitian, their main concern being that the level of catering skills varied enormously among staff. Some reported themselves or their peers to be excellent cooks and adept at budgeting in their own lives, while others openly admitted their limitations. However, regardless of skill level, staff and householders were expected to deliver a balanced, edible diet. In some cases, they were expected to enable people living in the house to do the same. Areas of operational practice that caused concern were encompassed in three main areas: practical cooking skills, menu planning and budgeting. The programme was organised as eight sessions, each of 7 hours, supported by tuition from the course tutors. The course ran over 8 weeks, with an additional minimum of 4 self-directed study days for student project work.

The aim of the course was that 'Participants will be able to meet the daily food and beverage needs of between three and eight clients through the provision of a range of nutritionally balanced and attractive meals by the preparation and cooking of a range of convenience, pre-prepared and fresh foods to meet budgetary targets and client requirements'.

A third of the course was spent in the kitchens on practical skills designed to meet NVQ level 1 (Hospitality and Catering), and a third in the classroom, covering menu planning, budgeting, nutrition and special dietary needs. Food safety was not formally part of the programme as a food handlers' certificate was a prerequisite. Projects formed another third of the course consolidating the knowledge and skills obtained. Each member of staff produced a 4-week menu specifically to meet the needs of the household in which they worked. Strict menu planning criteria and a budget of £2 (later increased) per person per day was set. The menu was then implemented by the member of staff and evaluated within 6–8 weeks of its commencement.

This course was piloted in April 1993, the evaluation of this project leading to further courses and the Regional Training Award of 1995. It demonstrated quality improvements in meals provided, clients' and staff's reactions were positive, and budgets were met. Additionally, staff motivation and interest were extremely high.

Seven courses have been run, with a total of 55 staff from learning disability services, three from mental health services. These have been run jointly with Highbury College of Further Education, which provides a professional, appropriate location and tuition. This joint partnership between education and health has provided support workers not only with a sense of achievement and being valued, but also with a qualification and new skills.

The course evaluation by the participants has been mostly positive, the exception being budgeting, which most people found difficult and boring. However, evaluation following implementation normally refutes previous negative statements about budgeting.

Staff acknowledge their skills responding with, 'Now I easily spot a good price.' The evaluation of their menu implementation occurs after each training course. Participants feed back the positive and negative aspects for the people in house, the staff and themselves. Common themes have been improved diets, more variety, good recipes, delicious food and a reduced time spent on shopping and considering menus. Mistakes have inevitably been made and, with each new course, gradually ironed out. The organisational audit will be completed in 1999.

Although it is neither a cheap nor a quick option, providers of small community houses should consider the benefits for staff training of using a course designed and run by people with the relevant professional skills.

Nutrition screening tools

An assessment of nutritional vulnerability is critical to providing an adequate diet. Two simple tools can form the foundation for assessment: a nutrition screening tool and a weight history. Weight histories are an important indicator of health. If a person or his or her carer cannot accurately reflect this history, important symptoms or health status may be missed.

A nutrition screening tool was developed with nursing staff and implemented in 1992, its aim being to screen people to ascertain their potential nutritional risk. The tool served two purposes: to refer on to a dietitian (if a person scored less than 8) and to act as a monitoring tool. It aimed to be repeated annually, thereby assessing whether a person's score had increased or decreased. Decreasing scores should result in questions ascertaining why the person was more at risk. The tool was purposely designed to be simple and quick for support workers to use and did not require nursing or dietetic input. Its use was aimed mainly at people still living in the hospital and integrated into the rehabilitation package.

The strengths of the tool were that the staff found it easy and quick to use, its limitation being its lack of formal validation. Nationally, few validated nutrition screening tools for any care group exist. Those which have undergone formal scrutiny are extremely clinical in nature and capture neither social nor emotional changes that may impact upon nutritional health. Two studies have aimed to validate the relevant screening tools. Bryan et al. (1998) have assessed the reliability and validity of a screening tool with adults living in a long-stay hospital for people with learning difficulties. In addition, a tool designed to be used for older people living in the community (Ward *et al.*, 1998) has not yet been reviewed for this group of people.

This Portsmouth screening tool was used in an audit prior to the closure of the long-stay hospital (Jukes *et al.*, 1994). The audit highlighted the use of the nutrition screening tool and weight records as an indicator. It demonstrated a high completion rate of screening tools but poor weight recording. The two standards audited relate specifically to nutritional health and were later incorporated into the division's Model of Care package.

These two indicators form the foundations of nutritional assessment; if used and systematically reviewed, they will identify a person nutritionally at risk. It is the author's opinion that nutrition screening and weight history indicators should be included in minimum nutrition standards. However, three service considerations arise prior to this development. Screening tools must be validated and appropriate to people's needs. Scales must also be available and appropriate for those people with physical disabilities. Debate should question whose role is it to carry out these activities: householders, unpaid carers, support workers, nurses or primary care teams?

Feeding people policy

Although publicity has arisen surrounding the nutritional status of patients in acute hospitals, few community health Trusts have audited or undertaken policy development in this area. Bradford Community Health NHS Trust has carried out an initial audit specifically looking at people's dietary needs. Its aim was 'To ensure clients receive a choice of a healthy well balanced diet and have their individual dietary needs identified and met' (Webster and Clark, 1995, p. 4). The auditor visited 20 houses and, using a minimum standards audit checklist, demonstrated that 11 houses scored 100 per cent. The key actions resulting from the audit were further staff training, the provision of recipes and an improved storage of food.

Portsmouth Healthcare NHS Trust has taken a strategic approach to this topic. A group of contract managers, representing all care groups (the Learning Disability Division, Elderly Mental Illness, Adult Mental Illness, Community Hospitals and Elderly

Medicine), the catering advisor, the dietitians and the Operational Director formed a working group to produce and implement a Feeding People policy over a 5-year period. It is totally supported by the Trust's Executive and is seen as one of the most crucial quality initiatives within the trust. The approach taken is novel in methodology as it follows a 5-year plan including training, resource development, policy development and audit. Minimum standards were developed using the DoH's guidelines and the checklist for audit (DoH, 1996). These were audited in 1997, selecting houses and wards from all care groups throughout the Trust.

Following the audit, one of the major actions was to identify a named person in each house or ward to become the nutrition representative. A training programme for these representatives commenced in 1998, including one from each of the 55 social and health care community houses in the Learning Disability Division. Their role is to form the crucial link between the working group, contract groups and house staff. Their initial training day focused upon minimum nutrition standards and identifying appropriate action plans for their own house. The representatives then discussed implementation with their staff groups and house managers. A feedback day identified their progress and also the barriers to change. The next stages are to reaudit and add to the minimum standards, enabling quality to spiral upwards in order to achieve comprehensive standards.

Quality spiral model

The audit spiral (Figure 11.1) suggests a diagramatic framework within which to develop nutrition standards. Although lengthy, it acknowledges the time constraints and endless demands placed upon service workers. However, it aims to skill and motivate people to provide high-quality food services. For those already doing so, the process demonstrates high standards and prevents complacency.

An audit spiral (Centre for Medical Education, 1995) may, however, be seen as too open – 'How do you know when to stop?' This will perhaps form a topic for future debate.

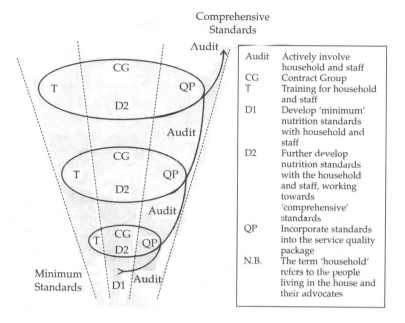

Figure 11.1   Nutrition standards: a spiral audit model

Conclusion

Food is close to most people's hearts, and it deserves the status attributed to it by most people in our society. Legislation states that people in registered care homes should be offered 'suitable, varied and properly prepared wholesome and nutritious food'. Nutrition standards may help define the meaning of these words. However, words alone are unlikely to have any impact unless householders and staff have the knowledge, skills and ownership to implement them. It must be remembered that most people with learning diffi-culties already experience little or no control over food issues in their life. Thus, nutrition standards should not dictate inflexible regimes but increase the enjoyment of food and enhance quality of life. This text has focused largely upon service provider involve-ment in this process, but the model needs to move onto stronger service user and purchaser involvement.

Checklist for action

- Nutrition standards can be a tool to measure national dietary targets.
- The nutritional needs of people who are underweight or over-active, or who have feeding difficulties, must be considered when applying dietary targets.
- The identification of people at nutritional risk requires a validated screening tool.
- Nutrition standards are necessary, but they should be facilitated rather than imposed.
- Minimum standards should initially be set, working towards comprehensive standards using a planned quality spiral model.
- Minimum standards should include screening and recording weight histories. Comprehensive standards will include all aspects of life relating to food.
- Nutritional standards should be integral to the organisation's service quality package.
- Audit should be self/peer group/user involvement led, and linked into systems such as the King's Fund organisational audit and the Registered Homes inspections.
- All health and social care – voluntary, private and statutory, residential accommodation – should be included.
- Service users should be both involved throughout the process and reap the benefits.

References

Ager, A. Working paper 1: Summary of preliminary findings regarding the use of the life experiences checklist as a measure of 'quality of life'. Unpublished paper. (Leicester: University of Leicester, 1986).

British Dietetic Association. *Mental Health Group: Profile on Dieticians Working for People with Learning Difficulties*. Unpublished, 1993.

British Dietetic Association. *Resource Pack: Nutrition Standards in Small Community Houses for People with Learning Difficulties*. (Birmingham: Mental Health Group, 2000).

Bryan, F., Jones, M. and Russel, L. 'Reliability and validity of a nutrition screening tool to be used with clients with learning disabilities.' *Journal of Human Nutrition and Dietetics*, 11(1998): 41–50.

Caudrey A. and Russell, O. 'Vitamin C status and dietary intake in a long stay unit for clients with learning disabilities: implications for community care.' *British Journal of Learning Disabilities*, 23(1995): 70–3.

Centre for Medical Education. *Moving to Audit: An Education Package for the Professions Allied to Medicine*. (Dundee: Postgraduate Office, Ninewells Hospital and Medical School, 1995).

Centre for Policy on Ageing. *Home Life: Code of Practice for Residential Care – Working Party Report*. (London: CPA, 1984).

Centre for Policy on Ageing. *A Better Home Life: Code of Good Practice for Residential and Nursing Home Care*. (London: CPA, 1996).

Cunningham, K., Gibney, M.J., Kelly, A., Kevany, J. and Mulcahy, M. 'Nutrient intakes in long-stay mentally handicapped persons.' *British Journal of Nutrition*, **64**(1990): 3–11.

Department of Health. *Nutrition Guidelines for Hospital Catering: A Checklist for Audit*. (Wetherby: DoH, 1996).

Department of Health and Human Services. *Medicaid Program: Conditions or Intermediate Care Facilities for the Mentally Retarded; Final Rule*. USA Federal Register: Part III, **53**(1988): 107.

Hay, F. and Jeffereys, K. A pilot study on the implementation strategies and monitoring of nutritional standards. Unpublished report. (Portsmouth: Portsmouth Healthcare Trust, 1992).

Jeffereys, K. An investigation into the current nutritional standards in seven small community houses for children and adults with learning disabilities in Portsmouth and South East Hampshire Health Authority. Unpublished MSc Research Study. (Portsmouth: University of Portsmouth, 1993).

Jukes, K., Jeffereys, K. and Wood, C. *Clinical Audit for Long Term Monitoring of Nutrition Status for Adults with a Learning Disability*. (Portsmouth: Portsmouth HealthCare NHS Trust, 1994).

King's Fund Audit. *Community, Mental Health and Learning Disabilities: Standards and Criteria*. (London: King's Fund, 1996).

Ministry of Health, Province of British Colombia. *Nutrition and Food Service Standards for Adult Care Facilities: Meal Management for Group Homes*. (Victoria, Canada: Queen's Printer, 1991).

National Development Group for Mentally Handicapped. *Improving the Quality of Services for Mentally Handicapped People: A Checklist of Standards*. (London: DHSS, 1980).

NHS Executive. *Hospital Catering: Delivering a Quality Service*. (Wetherby: DoH, 1996).

Royal College of Nursing. *Nutrition Standards and the Older Adult. RCN Dynamic Quality Improvement Programme*. (London: RCN, 1993).

Soneff, R. *Food Services Manual for Small Facilities*. (Canada: British Colombia Ministry of Health, 1991).

Soneff, R., McGeachy, F., Davidson, K., McCargar, L. and Therien, G. 'Effectiveness of two training methods to improve the quality of care in small facilities for adult care.' *Journal of the American Dietetic Association*, **8**(1994): 869–73.

Stewart, L., Beange, H. and Mackerras, D. 'A survey of dietary problems of adults with learning disabilities in the community.' *Mental Handicap Research*, **7**(1)(1994): 41–9.

Wallace, B. Nutrition in mental health residential services. Needs assessment: results. Unpublished report. (Australia: Northern Sydney Area Health Service, 1995).

Ward, J., Close, J., Boorman, J., Perkins, A., Cole S. and Edington, J. 'Development of a screening tool for assessing risk of undernutrition in patients in the community.' *Journal of Human Nutrition and Dietetics*, **11**(4)(1998): 323–30.

Webster D. and Clark, A. *An Initial Audit of Clients Dietary Needs.* Audit Summary. (Bradford: Bradford Community Health NHS Trust, Audit Department, 1995).

Whittacker, A., Gardener, S. and Kershaw J. *Service Evaluation by People with Learning Difficulties.* (London: King's Fund, 1991).

12
PREMISE FOR POSSIBILITIES

Roberta Astor

How to promote inclusion

This book has drawn together many different issues for people with learning difficulties. Although the topics are wide ranging, they address the underlying principles concerning equitable health services.

The chapters suggest areas for improving both health and social care. The authors have added to the existing knowledge base and recommended actions to be considered when promoting healthy lifestyles for people with learning difficulties. Their work complements two excellent documents, *Signposts for Success* (Lindsey, 1998) and *Building Expectations* (Mental Health Foundation, 1996). These documents make recommendations for good practice in all aspects of health and social care for people with learning difficulties. They derive advice directly from the experience of people with learning difficulties and their carers. Examples of both good and bad practice are given.

The use of recommendations made throughout this work will ensure that the rights of people with learning difficulties are recognised by the providers and purchasers of health and social health care. It also provides a firm foundation for quality assurance in both acute and primary health care.

The Health of the Nation: A Strategy for People with Learning Disabilities says that 'Education, social care and health cannot be easily separated' (DoH, 1995a, p. 10) and emphasises the importance of any 'health alliance', including 'general health services'.

The partnership anticipated by *The New NHS* (DoH, 1997) between health and social services, and the collaboration between primary care groups (PCGs) and NHS Trusts, leads to a positive expectation of improved health care for people with learning difficulties. A truly cooperative approach, in which health improvement is actively monitored, could iron out many present problems.

The Department of Health (DoH) has said:

New Primary Care Groups will be responsible for planning and developing services for smaller populations that will be sensitive to local health needs. Their contribution to drawing up and implementing Health Improvement Programmes will be vital, reflecting the perspective of the local community and building partnerships with key local organisations. (DoH, 1998, p. 41)

A major message given by the first chapter of this book is that health improvement programmes must actively assess and include the needs of people with learning difficulties.

The book shows the excellent work that a variety of professionals can do to promote health for people with learning difficulties. PCGs should access the expertise of professionals such as these.

Who can promote inclusion?

Building Expectations (Mental Health Foundation, 1996) recognises that it is unreasonable to expect all relevant professionals additionally to specialise in learning disabilities. However, it makes recommendations that 'all such specialists should gain familiarity in how to work with people with learning disabilities' (Mental Health Foundation, 1996, p. 61). Professionals specialising in this area are thin on the ground. It is also rare for professional health care education to contain much information to help them to work with people with learning difficulties.

The only health care educational curriculum that prepares professionals to specialise in working for people with learning difficulties is that of Registered Nurse for People with Learning Disabilities (RNLD). It seems essential, therefore, that learning disability nurses take influential roles in PCGs. Other disciplines of community nursing increasingly provide health care for people with learning difficulties. Their roles would be both strengthened and complemented by effective partnership with learning disability nurses. Health service guidelines (DoH, 1998) emphasise the importance of including community nurses in PCGs. With this membership, PCGs could provide excellent forums for improving and promoting the health of people with learning difficulties.

The Cullen Report sees health and social care as 'inextricably linked' and calls for 'harmony between health and social care skills in order to promote a measurable high quality service' (Chief Nursing Officers of the United Kingdom, 1991, p. 13) for people with learning difficulties. A major role is suggested for the learning disability nurse in promoting this harmony. The Report highlights that:

it is essential to have at least one group of staff whose theoretical and practical training is exclusively in mental handicap and who will therefore be better able to fulfil a generalist role precisely because they are also trained as specialists. For example, a nurse is equipped to be able to identify issues which might later become serious problems, such as the early signs of a psychiatric or physical condition, when these would not be obvious to an untrained person. Nurses carry out some tasks for which high level care skills are essential, and others where lower level skills are used, but knowledge of profound and multiple handicaps, other problems common in people with mental handicaps and of superimposed psychiatric conditions or behaviour disturbance enables better assessment, more effective focused rehabilitation work, earlier identification of ill health and more aggressive treatment of treatable conditions. (p. 6)

Building Expectations says:

It is important that GPs know which of their patients has a learning disability, so that steps can be taken to monitor their health care. (Mental Health Foundation, 1996, p. 58)

The role that a learning disability nurse can take, as part of a PCG, in supporting general practitioners (GPs) is shown by the following DoH case study:

General Practitioners in an area realised they had limited information concerning people on their lists who had learning disability. They also needed advice on their needs and the sorts of services available. One of the G.P.s contacted the Community Team and a Community Nurse visited. From the data base held in the team she was able to provide background information concerning the people on their lists and an outline of each person's needs. Together with the Practice Team it was decided that a more detailed assessment of need was required and the Community Nurse offered to devise a brief questionnaire which the G.P.s sent to parents for them to complete. The results were later analysed by the team and a plan constructed which included health screening and referral to specialists where necessary. All the people on the list now have regular screening for health-related problems, and conditions such as epilepsy are better managed. The Community Nurse now acts as a case manager for the people with learning disability on the list which has resulted in speedier referral for additional help. (DoH, 1995b, p. 11)

The United Kingdom Central Council for Nursing, Midwifery and Health Visiting (1997) describes the work of Karen Morgan, based in Surrey. The problems that people with learning difficulties had in accessing health services were recognised by the NHS Trust's executive nurse, Lesley Leach. She advocated a role for a clinical nurse specialist in primary care, who could specifically promote health care for people with learning difficulties. Leach describes Morgan's work as having no blueprint, adopting an unconventional role and possibly being the only one in the country. Her work is having a positive impact on health care for people with learning difficulties by informing them about healthy lifestyle issues and improving their access to health care.

There is no doubt that there is a strong case for giving learning disability nurses an important role in PCGs. This can be made by considering available information about the work they do to promote healthy lifestyles for people with learning difficulties. Kay *et al.* emphasised the ability of learning disability nurses to form an alliance with primary health care teams and work in partnership with other professionals (DoH, 1995b). Their work can be directly interactive with people and their carers or it can coordinate and guide the work of others. The argument for learning disability nurses taking this role is illustrated and reinforced by the following examples of learning disability nursing practice. Various personal details of clients described in these studies are changed to maintain confidentiality.

LIAISING WITH PRIMARY HEALTH CARE SERVICES:
A CASE STUDY BY CAROL HOLDEN,
COMMUNITY NURSE TEAM LEADER

Beth, a woman in her late forties, lives in residential accommodation with three other women. She receives 24-hour staff support and has been attending a local day centre. She would normally pursue a relatively full and active social life. She was referred to our team by the manager of her home

188

because she was experiencing faecal incontinence on a daily basis. This had increased over a number of months to the point where it interfered with every aspect of Beth's life.

My role, as a learning disability community nurse, was to coordinate the care given by other multidisciplinary professionals and untrained carers. By writing a care plan, I consolidated the involvement of everyone involved in Beth's care. I also used the care plan to guarantee that Beth was informed and involved by always consulting her about its content. I provided guidelines and support to ensure that everyone was following this care plan.

The care plan content was also discussed with Beth's direct carers. On occasion, I attended staff meetings, both at her house and at the day centre that she attends. This facilitated a decision making process regarding Beth's care. I also provided education about Beth's care and treatment.

Through regular meetings with Beth, supported by her staff team and in liaison with her GP, the following interventions were planned and implemented.

I familiarised myself with Beth's medical history and arranged to visit the GP with Beth and her residential keyworker. It transpired that Beth had a history of severe constipation and a previous diagnosis of megacolon. The GP had linked periods when Beth became confused and suffered a decline in mobility to the times when she was constipated. He thought that the toxins produced by constipation were having a severe effect on Beth's level of mental awareness. In order to prevent this, he had previously prescribed a daily dose of laxative (Manevac). Our combined discussion led to the conclusion that the dose of laxative, together with a poorly managed diet and insufficient fluid intake, was making it very difficult for Beth to control her bowels.

I arranged for bimonthly appointments of Beth, myself and her GP to review and gradually reduce the dosage of laxative medication. I helped the staff team to monitor Beth's bowel actions and developed their ability to observe the symptoms of constipation, as experienced by Beth. These were a decline in mobility, flatulence, an extended abdomen and a decline in her level of mental alertness. We arranged for the district nurse to visit whenever staff suspected that Beth was becoming constipated. She carried out a rectal examination and administered a suppository, which was now prescribed for Beth, if required. I was unable to administer the suppository as my learning disability team were not contracted by the local health authority to provide a clinical service that could be provided by primary health care services.

I liaised with the dietitian, who assisted me in providing advice and guidance about healthy eating to Beth and her staff. This focused on promoting Beth's general health and preventing her becoming constipated. Information was given about menu planning for a healthy diet, as well as advice on how to identify the effect of certain foods on Beth's bowels. A definite link was made between her eating these foods and having periods of faecal incontinence. The staff were also educated in enabling Beth to maintain an adequate fluid intake. They were informed about the necessity of a minimum daily fluid intake, the types of fluid to either encourage or avoid and the ways in which this could affect health. I worked with Beth, her staff and the dietitian to produce guidelines covering all of these issues. Beth received positive support from her staff, which encouraged her involvement in this process.

I contacted the occupational therapist and physiotherapist for guidance about assessing Beth's mobility. I made initial joint visits to Beth, with both therapists. They carried out assessments and provided reports. I assisted Beth's staff team in incorporating the contents of these reports into her care plan. The main outcomes of this intervention were the provision of walking aids (a range of which were tried over a period of time), a wheelchair for use out of the house, when Beth's mobility was particularly poor, and a passive exercise programme. The physiotherapist was actively involved in monitoring the exercise programme and updating it according to need.

The main focus of the care plan centred on the promotion of positive bowel management for Beth. This included:

- monitoring, through accurate record keeping, all bowel movements and all incidents of faecal incontinence;
- menu planning and monitoring of her diet;
- ensuring an adequate fluid intake;
- providing regular opportunities for active and passive exercise;
- ensuring a rapid response to the signs and symptoms of constipation by providing a step-by-step guide of the action to be taken should constipation be suspected;
- regular reviews, together with Beth's GP, of the medication prescribed for her bowel management.

I assisted the staff team in analysing the information gathered by their recording systems on a regular basis, updating the care plan accordingly.

The most effective and crucial intervention in this whole programme of care was the regular meetings with the GP. Once he recognised the extent and value of my role, he proved very supportive. Prior to my involvement, he had little awareness of the effect on Beth of a large dose of laxative, coupled with poor bowel control. I brought this to his attention, and we jointly agreed interventions to address the problem. We always met in Beth's presence. I usually accompanied her to the surgery, and she was involved at all times as the focus of our planning.

By giving guidelines and monitoring the care planning process, I provided evaluated information on Beth's current health. This gave the GP a sound foundation on which to base his medical decisions. I was able to identify possible causes of both Beth's constipation and faecal incontinence, suggest treatments and clarify my thought processes through discussion with the GP.

Although Beth is still not completely continent, a positive bowel management care plan has currently been implemented to good effect. Beth can have several weeks at a time free from faecal incontinence. She has resumed all of her social activities, and her health is very well monitored. She still has glycerine suppositories prescribed, to be used as necessary, but these are now a last resort. The staff team's raised awareness of Beth's condition means that we can respond promptly to any suspicion of constipation, thus avoiding the unnecessary administration of the suppositories.

ACCESSING DENTAL CARE IN THE COMMUNITY
BY KATHRYN CURTIS, TEAM LEADER RESIDENTIAL SERVICES

Our service provides care in the community and aims to meet specific health care needs for clients who have severe learning difficulties. We try to ensure that all routine preventive treatment is carried out, including dental checks and care.

Approaching local dental surgeries was out of the question as they considered our service to be under the 'umbrella' of hospital care. In addition, surgery facilities would not have been suitable for the wheelchairs belonging to our clients. Because of the nature of clients' disabilities, these wheelchairs tend to be twice the length of an average wheelchair. The situation was not helped by the shortage of dentists willing to admit NHS patients to their lists.

We therefore approached the local dental clinic and were delighted with the response and care given. This is partly because of the dental surgeon and his staff. They always talk directly to the client and involve us in the conversation. They direct questions to the client, although they are aware that the client can not communicate verbally. They ensure eye contact and are careful in the positioning of their bodies. They are willing to make two or three appointments to get to know the client and they make house calls when appropriate. They never make us feel rushed and always respond positively to our questions. They respond promptly to client needs and make sure that there is no long wait for treatment.

We often find that other professionals are uneasy with people who have severe learning difficulties. It was impressive to meet people who are natural and whose manner is irreproachable.

A CASE WHERE THE LEARNING DISABILITY NURSE COULD HAVE HELPED
BY AMANDA YERBURY, COMMUNITY LEARNING DISABILITY NURSE

I met Ann after she had been admitted to an acute general hospital from private sector residential accommodation. Her initial diagnosis was of an acute medical condition requiring bed rest and medication. This treatment was given until it was discovered that her real problem was constipation. Ann also has mental health needs.

Hospital staff overestimated Ann's self-help skills. They had left her tablets on the bedside locker, which meant that she had not been taking her prescribed antipsychotic medication. Because of this and the effects of constipation, she became very confused and did not drink (fluid also having been left on the bedside table). Ann's condition so concerned her residential staff that they felt unable to take her home on discharge as they did not think that she was physically or mentally well enough. They asked for intervention from learning disability services, and Ann was referred to me. I visited Ann in hospital and concurred with the opinion of her residential staff. I noticed that Ann's fluid chart indicated that urine had not been passed for 24 hours.

Unfortunately, the hospital insisted upon discharging Ann. She was discharged to an NHS assessment unit for people with learning difficulties as she was not well enough to return home. This was an unnecessary crisis response rather than appropriate action to take for Ann.

Had Ann been referred to me earlier, perhaps before her admission to hospital, I could have provided an effective link between her staff and acute care staff. It is probable I could even have prevented her admission in the first place. As Ann's GP organised her admission to hospital, I think that this illustrates the need for primary health care staff to talk to learning disability community nurses.

GETTING THE RIGHT SERVICE: A GRADUAL PROGRESSION
BY AMANDA YERBURY

Carol is in her forties; she has a moderate learning difficulty. When I first met Carol, she still lived at home with her elderly mother, Mrs Arnold. Carol's father had died 10 years previously, and since his death, Carol rarely went out, except to attend a day centre. Carol's mother enjoyed an active social life, which Carol declined invitations to share. Carol also refused offers of respite care to allow her mother a holiday.

Four years ago, a social worker referred Carol to a consultant psychiatrist for people with learning difficulties. The referral was made because Carol was attacking clients and staff at her day centre. As Carol is a large strong woman, these attacks resulted in serious physical injuries.

The consultant diagnosed Carol as having paranoid schizophrenia. This diagnosis was based on Carol expressing feelings of persecution and stating that she heard voices making derogatory personal remarks. She thought that people were talking about her, plotting against her and making death threats towards her. The consultant found interviewing Carol like walking on thin ice as she obviously felt so threatened. Meetings to review Carol's care had added to her paranoia as they confirmed the idea that people were talking about her.

Carol's GP had prescribed a low dose of thoridazine, a major tranquilliser. The consultant agreed with this prescription and recommended its continuation. Carol did not like taking it as she feared it would turn her into a 'drug addict', and Carol's mother reinforced this. She did not consider the medication suitable for Carol, and she did not agree with anyone taking medication unnecessarily. Unfortunately, Carol's GP had not explained her illness to either her or her mother and had described the medication as 'knockout tablets'.

Carol's behaviour had definitely challenged people at the day centre. She was consequently referred to a learning disability community nursing team specialising in care for people who exhibit 'challenging behaviour'. A community nurse went to the day centre to observe Carol. This caused Carol to think that she was being watched, so she hid in the ladies' toilet, and no observations could be recorded.

It was recognised that a community nurse with competence in both learning disabilities and mental health would be the appropriate practitioner for Carol, and this was where I came in.

I introduced myself to Mrs Arnold. She had previously been wary of any contact with health or social service professionals and had never met a community nurse before. Mrs Arnold appeared welcoming, and I felt able to build a mutually respectful rapport with her. I helped her to gain an understanding of Carol's condition. This insight shocked her as she considered that there was a stigma attached to having a mental illness. I explained how Carol's symptoms resulted from a neurological chemical imbalance that could be corrected by medication. I told Mrs Arnold that the brain was just one of the body's organs that could cause health problems, in the same way that a malfunctioning pancreas can cause someone to be diabetic and therefore need insulin. She was able to accept this.

I explained to Carol that taking her medication would help her to feel calmer and reduce her problem of hearing voices, which upset her so much. I gave Mrs Arnold a weekly dosette box, both to help her to ensure that Carol's medication intake was correct and to aid Carol towards independence through self-medication.

I initially visited weekly to assess Carol's symptoms and response to the medication. I asked Carol how she was feeling, whether the voices had been bothering her and what she was doing at the day centre. I thought it important that Carol should not be ashamed of her feelings or symptoms and that she could discuss them freely.

I liaised closely with the day centre. No baseline reading of Carol's behaviour had been taken, but recorded monitoring was taking place. Areas of Carol's behaviour that were monitored were her participation in activities, incidents of physical or verbal aggression, her appearance and her attendance.

Over a 2-week period, Carol became more relaxed. She said that she had not recently heard voices. Carol's appearance improved; she became warm and friendly and demonstrated a sense of humour. I reminded Carol that her medication was helping her. At the day centre, it was observed that Carol had dramatically increased her participation in activities and was also much less verbally aggressive.

Carol was beginning to take responsibility for her medication. She would remind her mother when medication was due and had started to put tablets in the dosette box for herself. After 3 months, when Carol was stable and progressing, I began to decrease the frequency of my visits, gradually reducing my input to a monthly visit. I would sometimes visit Carol and her mother at home and sometimes Carol at the day centre.

Carol remained stable for a year and then relapsed, of which I became aware when I visited her at home. She was very hostile, slamming doors and swearing. I decided that it was best not to confront Carol and opted to sit down and have a cup of tea with her mother. Mrs Arnold said she was frightened and worried about Carol. Although a year was the longest period of stability she could remember Carol having, this relapse surprised her. I reassured Mrs Arnold that relapses were not unusual and that they were only

193

temporary. After half an hour, Carol joined us for a cup of tea. She apologised for her behaviour, saying that she hoped she had not frightened me; I had taken care not to appear frightened. However, when Carol asked, I admitted that I had been frightened and was surprised and worried about what could be upsetting her. Carol said that she was being talked about at the day centre and that someone had tried to poison her.

I checked with the day centre to make sure Carol's beliefs were not real, before concluding that her mental health had deteriorated. I alerted Carol's doctors, who changed her medication to Risperalal. Carol responded positively to this change. She became more helpful at home and good company for her mother. She did not report hearing voices. At the day centre, Carol's mood was reported as stable and tolerant towards other people. Social services employed an additional person to work with Carol, the aim being to increase her socialisation and participation in activities. The person gradually gained Carol's trust and respect. Consequently, Carol participated in cookery, music and craft sessions.

Carol continued to refuse respite care. However, as Mrs Arnold now always enjoyed her daughter's company, this did not seem to present a problem.

Following Carol's relapse, I had increased the frequency of my visits to weekly, again alternating these between her home and the day centre. Carol's initial prescribed dose of Risperalal was low. The dose was increased to titration level in small doses over time. As Carol stabilised again, I phased out my visits to once every 3 weeks; this took 3 months.

Then, on a visit to the day centre, I noticed that Carol looked ill. She was pale, lethargic and breathless, and her personal hygiene had deteriorated. I contacted Carol's mother to discuss this. Mrs Arnold reported that Carol was ill and had recurrent diarrhoea. She suggested this was caused by a lack of fresh air because Carol so rarely went out. I suggested that Carol should go to her GP and have a blood test. Mrs Arnold said she would arrange this, but I did not wholly believe her.

I shared my concerns about Carol with the consultant psychiatrist and hoped that Carol would go to the GP. After a fortnight, I visited Carol's home again. Mrs Arnold was still suggesting that a lack of fresh air was Carol's problem and had not taken her to the GP. I suggested arranging for the GP's practice nurse to visit Carol at home for the blood test. Mrs Arnold remained reluctant. I informed the consultant psychiatrist, who decided to visit Carol at the day centre and then liaise with her GP.

Before this visit happened, Mrs Arnold telephoned me asking whether I could come urgently as Carol was ill. I told her to contact the GP and that I was on my way. On arrival, I found Mrs Arnold and Carol's two sisters in a very distressed state. I went to see Carol, who was in bed. At first she appeared not to recognise me. She was pale and said she had a severe headache and was unsteady on her feet. I took her pulse and temperature, which were normal. The GP arrived. He did not consider Carol ill enough to need hospital admission, but arranged for blood tests to be taken the next day. I contacted Carol's consultant psychiatrist, who advised that the Risperalal should be stopped. I arranged this and then explained about blood tests to Carol.

The next day Mrs Arnold telephoned me again, she said that Carol had deteriorated and that she could not cope. She asked me to come, and I immediately contacted the GP, who arranged Carol's admission to an acute care hospital. I stayed with Carol and her mother until the ambulance arrived. One of Carol's sisters went to hospital with her. The sister later told me that Carol was questioned on admission to hospital. She was asked the date, where she was, how old she was and the name of the Prime Minister. Carol got the answers wrong so they had her transferred to a hospital for people with mental health problems, where I visited her the next day. The registrar had examined Carol. Examination revealed Carol to be suffering from chest infection, severe constipation, urinary tract infection and suspected anaemia. Arrangements were being made to transfer her back to the acute care hospital.

Carol was admitted to the appropriate hospital and successfully treated for her many illnesses. During this hospital stay, I took the opportunity to suggest residential care for Carol to her mother, and Mrs Arnold agreed. A social worker took Mrs Arnold and Carol's sisters to look at various residential homes. They chose a home with a good record of caring for people who had needs like Carol's. I regularly visited Carol in hospital, but it was decided that her sisters would tell her about the residential home plans.

On first hearing the news that her mother was no longer able to look after her at home, Carol was understandably upset. Carol's family said they would always visit her and that she could go and visit her mother.

When Carol was well enough, I took her to the residential home for tea. She was talkative and enjoyed meeting the other people who lived there, some of whom she knew from the day centre. After seeing her bedroom, Carol agreed to stay for a trial period.

Carol has now been happily living in her new home for a year. Her care is monitored monthly. She regularly takes a taxi to visit her mother, has made new friends and seems very content. I still occasionally visit to keep in touch.

Why promote inclusion?

Governments and industry frequently take actions or make safety errors that endanger health globally. Positive health behaviour stems from informed choice and statutory protection from abuse, health being a basic human right. It can be difficult for many people to choose positive health behaviour because of a lack of resources and information. Most of us are denied the right to make informed choices about what we eat as a result of the food industry's unwillingness to label foodstuffs simply, despite the DoH's pledge to 'ensure that the public and others have the information they need to improve their health' (DoH, 1998, p. 30). This example extends into other areas of health behaviour as a result of various political, professional and private vested interests.

It can be hoped that people have a level of awareness about what they do not know. This awareness will help them to seek and lobby for information with which to inform their lifestyle choices. This is not so for people with moderate or severe learning difficulties, particularly if they also have sensory or physical disabilities. Their concentration span and cognitive or physical ability may not be sufficient to allow them access to available health information.

Professionals and informal carers working to promote health with people who have these disabilities will frequently invent good teaching resources and strategies. Unless these are publicised, they are lost to others who could use them. There should be the means for collecting these ideas and resources, and making them available nationally. The Health Education Authority (HEA) has attempted this; their efforts should be expanded and their resources made publicly available.

Similarly, there should be a means of the national dissemination of information about good professional practice, which ensures access to appropriate health care. The first chapter of this book emphasises the need for publicly available local and national information networks that include examples of good practice. Currently available networks such as the English National Board for Nursing, Midwifery and Health Visiting (ENB) and the HEA do make some information available. The ENB aims to provide a range of useful information, including 'Specialist practice area information (currently sadly lacking in Learning Disability Information – a problem which could soon be tackled by the ("network")' (ENB, 1998, p. 1).

We must remain aware that while society may view people with learning difficulties as 'incurable', this can determine the health promotion and health care approach that is adopted. Pitfalls in community care and health service delivery remain – they will not disappear if services are underresourced.

Positive change has begun. Innovations in care and service direction are increasing, and the emphasis of research has dramatically changed. It no longer aims to discover new syndromes with which to label people; instead, syndromes have become conditions to take into account as part of health care. A pattern of research has arrived that seeks to enhance the life chances of people with learning difficulties, and importantly is sometimes directly participatory with potential service users. People with learning difficulties are increasingly speaking out for their rights. The choice of a healthy lifestyle is a fundamental human right. The arena of influence on health is one in which everyone's voice should be heard.

References

Chief Nursing Officers of the United Kingdom. *Caring for People: The Implications for Mental Handicap Nursing.* The Cullen Report. (London: DoH, 1991).

Department of Health. *The Health of the Nation: A Strategy for People with Learning Disabilities.* (London: HMSO, 1995a).

Department of Health. *Learning Disability: Meeting Needs Through Targeting Skills.* (London: DoH, 1995b).

Department of Health. *The New NHS, Modern, Dependable.* (London: Stationery Office, 1997).

Department of Health. *Our Healthier Nation, A Contract for Health: A Consultative Paper.* (London: Stationery Office, 1998).

English National Board for Nursing, Midwifery and Health Visiting. *Widening the Network with the World Wide Web.* National Network Newsletter. (London: ENB, 1998).

Kay, B., Rose, S. and Turnbull, J. *Continuing the Commitment: The Report of the Learning Disability Nursing Project.* (London: DoH, 1995).

Lindsey, M. *Signposts for Success in Commissioning and Providing Health Services for People with Learning Disabilities.* (Wetherby: DoH, 1998).

Mental Health Foundation. *Building Expectations: Opportunities and Services for People with a Learning Disability.* (London: Mental Health Foundation, 1996).

UKCC. *Scope in Practice.* (London: UKCC, 1997).

INDEX

multidisciplinary approach, to
  children's sleep problems 144–5
multisectoral collaboration 22
mumps, and hearing loss 118
music
  and exercise 40, 40–1
  and relaxation 42
myopia 101

N

National Curriculum, inclusion of sex
  education 56
National Health Service and
  Community Care Act 1990 4, 154, 162
National Plate Model 16, 43
National Vocational Qualifications
  (NVQs) 11–12, 33
neighbourhoods, healthy 13–14
  and healthy living centres 35
neonatal factors, and hearing loss
  118–19
neuromuscular tension control
  relaxation programme 41
New Jersey, USA, developmental
  disabilities centre 27
The New NHS (DoH document) 5, 6, 7,
  185
New Zealand, nutrition standards 173
nightmares 139
  v. night (sleep) terrors 140–1
night (sleep) terrors 140
  v. nightmares 140–1
night-time attacks (parasomnias)
  139–41
'nurturing', in RESPOND model 63
nutrition
  and eye vulnerability 103
  food labelling, symbolic 15–16, 44
  impacting on health 21
  research 173–6
  risk of being nutritionally
    compromised 165
  screening tools 178–9
  see also diet; nutrition standards
nutritional health, and nutrition
  standards 167
nutrition standards 165–84
  in acute hospitals 166
  aims 168
  audit 170–1, 179–80, 180–1
  checklist for action 182
  definition 167
  and environment 167
  food quality 167
  imposition *v.* negotiation in
    implementation of 173–4

independence 167
international perspective 171–3
key areas 167
King's Fund 170–1
national perspective 169–71
need for? 167–8
nutritional health 167
Registered Homes Act 1984 169–70
research study 174–6
self-advocacy 167
see also diet; food; Portsmouth
  Healthcare NHS Trust
Nutrition Task Force 16, 43

O

obstructive sleep apnoea 138, 141, 143
oppression, historical 69, 70, 75
optic atrophy 101
orientation, in visual impairment, *see*
  mobility and orientation
otitis media, *see* secretory otitis media
  (glue ear)
Our Healthier Nation (DoH document) 5,
  66
  healthy neighbourhoods 13–14, 35
  healthy schools 11–12
  healthy workplaces 12–13
  key health targets 7, 10–11, 112
  targeted groups 7–8

P

parasomnias (night-time attacks)
  139–41
parenting
  professional awareness of 79
  research 81
  rights 82
participation, of service users 69
participatory dialogue 71, 75, 76, 77
  case studies and discussion on 71–7
  effect on staff 76
partnership models, *see* antenatal care;
  residential settings
passivity 57
perinatal factors, and hearing loss 118
PIC sums 84
placing out technique, in relaxation 41
Portsmouth Healthcare NHS Trust,
  nutrition strategy 176–81
  audit spiral 180–1
  catering skills courses 176–8
  feeding people policy 179–80
  nutritional representatives 180
  nutrition screening tools 178–9
  weight histories 178–9
postnatal infection, and hearing loss 118